Earn CME credits while yc

Up to 75 *AMA PRA Category 1 Credits*™ available with the MedStudy 2010 Pediatrics Board-Style Questions & Answers

MedStudy is accredited by the Accreditation Council for Continuing Medical Education to provide continuing medical education for physicians.

MedStudy designates this educational activity for a maximum of 75 *AMA PRA Category 1 Credits*™. Physicians should only claim credit commensurate with the extent of their participation in the activity.

To receive CME credit, you must complete the **CME Credit Application** and **evaluation** found on the following pages, and then submit these along with the $40 CME processing fee to MedStudy. All the necessary contact information is included on the Application form.

Please note: CME credit is available **only** to the **original** purchaser of this product, and issuance of CME credit is subject to verification of product ownership.

The release date for the 2010 Pediatrics Board-Style Questions & Answers is January 1, 2010. To be eligible for CME credit, you must study the content of this activity and submit your CME application form no later than **January 1, 2013**.

LEARNING OBJECTIVES

As a result of participation in this activity, learners will be able to:

- Integrate and demonstrate increased overall knowledge of Pediatrics

- Identify and remedy areas of weakness (gaps) in knowledge and clinical competencies

- Describe the clinical manifestations and treatments of diseases encountered in Pediatrics and effectively narrow the differential diagnosis list by utilizing the most appropriate medical studies

- Apply the competence and confidence gained through participation in this activity to both a successful Board exam-taking experience and daily practice

Target Audience / Method of Participation

Participants in this educational activity are those physicians interested in expanding their knowledge in Pediatrics, focusing their learning on subjects that are directly relevant to clinical scenarios and associated questions that will be encountered on the ABP Board certifying or recertifying (MoC) exam.

Use the question-answer content as a self-study, self-testing exercise, attempting to answer questions as though they are part of an actual Board exam. Compare your selected answers against the answers given as "correct" in the Answer Book to assess your level of knowledge and recall of pertinent medical facts and clinical decision-making. Review your results to see your relative strengths and weaknesses by topic areas. Repeat the self-testing process as often as necessary to improve your knowledge and proficiency and ultimately to ensure your mastery of the material.

2010 PEDIATRICS MEDICINE BOARD-STYLE
QUESTIONS & ANSWERS

DISCLOSURE SUMMARY

It is the policy of MedStudy to ensure balance, independence, objectivity, and scientific rigor in all of its educational materials. All contributors participating in this program have disclosed to MedStudy any potential conflicts of interest related to the content they have provided. This pertains to any affiliation with an entity producing, marketing, re-selling, or distributing health care goods or services consumed by, or used on, patients. These disclosures are documented below, and any perceived conflicts of interest have been identified and resolved by MedStudy's CME Physicians Oversight Council prior to publication.

I. The following contributors have indicated affiliation with organizations that have interests which may relate to content they have provided:

Contributor	Affiliation	Name of Organization
Sara Copeland, MD	Grant/Research Support	BioMarin
	Consultant	Genzyme

II. The following contributors have documented they have nothing to disclose:

Moira Pfeifer, MD	Donald Beam, MD	Mark Corkins, MD, CNSP, FAAP
Thomas Krzmarzick, MD	Sriram S. Narsipur, MD	E. Ann Yeh, MD, FRCP(C)
Keith Boyd, MD	Daniel Polk, MD	Breck Nichols, MD, MPH
Amy Jo Nopper, MD	Arthur Pickoff, MD	Kimberly Jones, MD
Paul Catalana, MD, MPH		

III. The following contributors have received requests but have not provided disclosure information: None

IV. Good Practices Agreement: All contributors have signed a Good Practices Agreement affirming that their content is based upon currently available, scientifically rigorous data; that the content is free from commercial bias; and that clinical practice and patient care recommendations presented in the content are based on the best available evidence for these specialties and subspecialties.

MedStudy presents this activity for educational purposes only. Material is prepared based on multiple sources of information, but content is not intended to be exhaustive of the subject matter. Participants are expected to utilize their own expertise and judgment while engaged in the practice of medicine.

V. MedStudy Disclosure

MedStudy Corporation, including all of its employees, **does not** have a financial interest, arrangement, or affiliation with any commercial organization that may have a direct or indirect interest in the content presented in this activity. This includes any entity producing, marketing, re-selling, or distributing health care goods or services consumed by, or used on, patients. Furthermore, MedStudy complies with the AMA Council on Ethical and Judicial Affairs (CEJA) opinions that address the ethical obligations that underpin physician participation in CME: 8.061, "Gifts to physicians from industry," and 9.011, "Continuing Medical Education."

Author / Contributors — 2010 Pediatrics Board-Style Q&As

Author/Editor

J. Thomas Cross, Jr., MD, MPH, FAAP
Vice President – Education
Activity Director, 2010 Pediatrics Board-Style Questions & Answers
Member, MedStudy's CME Physicians Oversight Council
MedStudy Corporation
Colorado Springs, CO

Contributors

Donald Beam, MD
Director, Sickle Cell Program
Pediatric Hematology/Oncology
Cook Children's Medical Center
Fort Worth, TX

Keith Boyd, MD
Associate Chair for Education
Department of Pediatrics
Rush University Medical Center
Chicago, IL

Paul Catalana, MD, MPH
Professor of Clinical Pediatrics
Assistant Dean for Medical Education
University of South Carolina School of Medicine
Greenville, SC

Sara Copeland, MD
Clinical Assistant Professor, Pediatrics
Division of Medical Genetics / Department of Pediatrics
University of Iowa Children's Hospital
Medical Director, Iowa Neonatal Metabolic Screening
Iowa City, IA

Mark Corkins, MD, CNSP, FAAP
Associate Professor of Clinical Pediatrics
Indiana University School of Medicine
Division of Gastroenterology/Hepatology/Nutrition
Riley Hospital for Children
Indianapolis, IN

Kimberly Jones, MD
Associate Professor, Pediatrics and Medicine
Section Chief, Pediatrics Pulmonary
Department of Pulmonary Medicine
Louisiana State University Health Sciences Center
Shreveport, LA

Thomas Krzmarzick MD
Medical Director, Emergency Department
The Children's Medical Center
Dayton, OH

Sriram S. Narsipur, MD
Associate Professor of Medicine and Pediatrics
Nephrology Division
SUNY Upstate Medical University
Syracuse, NY

Breck Nichols, MD, MPH
Assistant Professor, Division of Allergy/Immunology
Director, Medicine and Pediatrics Residency Program
Los Angeles County Medical Center + University of Southern
California School of Medicine
Los Angeles, CA

Amy Jo Nopper, MD
Chief, Section of Dermatology
Children's Mercy Hospital
Kansas City, MO

Moira Pfeifer, MD
Pediatric Endocrinologist
The Children's Medical Center
Dayton, OH

Arthur S. Pickoff, MD
Professor and Chair
Department of Pediatrics
The Children's Medical Center / Wright State University
Dayton, OH

Daniel Polk, MD
Professor of Pediatrics
Northwestern University Medical School
Chief, Division of Hospital-based Medicine
Children's Memorial Hospital
Chicago, IL

E. Ann Yeh, MD, FRCP(C)
Assistant Professor of Neurology
Division of Child Neurology
SUNY at Buffalo
Clinical Co-Director, Pediatric MS Center
Jacobs Neurological Institute
Buffalo, NY

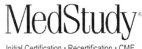

Initial Certification • Recertification • CME

P.O. Box 38148
Colorado Springs, CO 80937-8148
Phone: 1-800-841-0547
FAX: 1-719-520-5973

CME CREDIT APPLICATION

IMPORTANT: You must complete this form and submit it (and the evaluation) to MedStudy to receive CME credit. CME credit is available <u>only</u> to the original purchaser of this product. Issuance of a CME Certificate is subject to verification of product ownership.

CME Credit Application
2010 Pediatrics Board-Style Questions & Answers (Books)

MedStudy is accredited by the Accreditation Council for Continuing Medical Education (ACCME) to provide continuing medical education for physicians.

MedStudy designates this educational activity for a maximum of 75 *AMA PRA Category 1 Credits™*. Physicians should only claim credit commensurate with the extent of their participation in the activity.

The release date for the 2010 Pediatrics Board-Style Questions & Answers is January 1, 2010.
To be eligible for CME credit, you must study the content of these books and submit your CME credit application form no later than **January 1, 2013**.

My signature on this document certifies my participation in this MedStudy CME activity (one hour = one credit).

I am claiming _____ *AMA PRA Category 1 Credits™* (maximum credits: 75).

Signature:_____ **Date**: _____

Printed Name: _____

Street Address: _____

City/State/Zip Code:_____

Telephone: _____ Fax: _____

Permanent E-mail*:_____

Exact name of **original purchaser** (individual or institution) ☐ Same as above ☐ Other_____

Please select the method of delivery for your completed CME certificate. (*E-mail preferred.)

_____Mail _____Fax _____**E-mail** (Please ensure that your e-mail will accept PDF attachments from MedStudy.)

CME processing fee: $40

Payment method: __ Check or money order (payable to MedStudy); mail to address above

__ Visa __ MasterCard; FAX to: **(719) 520-5973** (include credit card information)

Card # _____ Expiration Date _____

Authorized Signature on Credit Card Account _____

Please print credit card name if different from applicant:_____

Please print billing address of card if different from above.   Street or P O Box: _____

City/State/Zip: _____

Continued on next page

IMPORTANT: EVERY question on this Evaluation MUST be answered.
2010 Pediatrics Board-Style Q&As

Affiliation: ☐ Practicing M.D. ☐ Practicing D.O. ☐ Resident/Fellow ☐ Non-Physician

Specialty: ☐ Peds ☐ IM/Peds ☐ Other: _____

How did you hear about this product?
☐ Catalog ☐ Colleague ☐ MedStudy Website ☐ Internet Search ☐ Medical Meeting ☐ Other

Which of the following BEST describes your use of this product?
☐ Prepare for Initial **Certification** ☐ Prepare for **Recertification** (MoC) ☐ **General Review/Reference**

When did you most recently take (or will you take) your ABP exam? Year_____ Month_____

Did you pass the ABP exam? ☐ Yes ☐ No ☐ Don't know yet ☐ Haven't taken it yet ☐ Didn't use product for exam prep

On a scale of 1 to 5, with 1 being STRONGLY DISAGREE and 5 being STRONGLY AGREE, please rate (and circle) the following regarding your use of this product:

	STRONGLY DISAGREE				STRONGLY AGREE

Due to my learning with this product, I am able to...

Integrate and demonstrate increased overall knowledge of Pediatrics	1	2	3	4	5
Identify and remedy areas of weaknesses (gaps) in knowledge and clinical competencies	1	2	3	4	5
Describe the clinical manifestations and treatments of diseases encountered in Pediatrics and effectively narrow the differential diagnosis list by utilizing the most appropriate medical studies	1	2	3	4	5
Apply the competence and confidence gained through participation in this activity to both a successful Board exam-taking experience and daily practice	1	2	3	4	5
The content presented met my personal educational expectations	1	2	3	4	5
Question and Answer exercise format was a viable mode of instructional delivery	1	2	3	4	5
The content was free of pharmaceutical bias	1	2	3	4	5
The content offered a reasonable balance of diagnostic and therapeutic options	1	2	3	4	5

Please rate the quality of coverage for the following specialty/subspecialty areas:

	POOR		FAIR		EXCELLENT
Adolescence	1	2	3	4	5
Allergy / Immunology / Rheumatology	1	2	3	4	5
Cardiology	1	2	3	4	5
Dermatology	1	2	3	4	5
Emergency Medicine	1	2	3	4	5
Endocrinology	1	2	3	4	5
ENT / Ophthalmology / Orthopedics	1	2	3	4	5
Gastroenterology	1	2	3	4	5
Genetics / Metabolic Disease	1	2	3	4	5
Growth & Development	1	2	3	4	5
Health Supervision	1	2	3	4	5
Hematology / Oncology	1	2	3	4	5
Infectious Disease	1	2	3	4	5
Nephrology	1	2	3	4	5
Nervous System / Neurology	1	2	3	4	5
Newborn / Prenatal Care	1	2	3	4	5
Nutrition / Teeth	1	2	3	4	5
Respiratory	1	2	3	4	5

In using this product, did you rectify practice knowledge gaps you were aware of—or identify knowledge gaps you had not been aware of?

☐ Yes
☐ No

If yes, please elaborate:

Were there specific topic areas that you encountered on the Board exam that you feel were not adequately covered in this product?

☐ Yes
☐ No
☐ Have not taken the exam

If yes, please elaborate:

The **most** valuable aspects of this product were:

General comments about this product or the ABP Board exam

Thank you for completing this Evaluation.
Please return this evaluation, along with your CME Credit Application, to MedStudy.

MedStudy®

Pediatrics Board-Style Questions & Answers

Questions

Edited by J. Thomas Cross, Jr., MD, MPH, FAAP

TABLE OF CONTENTS

Note: Many of the images you see throughout this Questions book can be viewed in color in the image atlas at the back of the book.

NOTICE: THESE BOOKS ARE MEANT TO BE USED AS AN ADJUNCT TO THE MEDSTUDY CORE CURRICULUM. THE PEDIATRIC BOARDS COVER A VAST REALM OF INFORMATION, AND BOARD SIMULATION QUESTIONS ALONE SHOULD NOT BE YOUR ONLY PREPARATION FOR THE BOARDS!

A NOTE ON EDITORIAL STYLE: There is an ongoing debate in medical publishing about whether to use the possessive form that adds " 's " to the names of diseases and disorders, such as Lou Gehrig's disease, Klinefelter's syndrome, and others. We acknowledge there is not a unanimous consensus on this style convention, but we think it is important to be consistent in what style we choose. For this publication, we have dropped the possessive form. The *AMA Manual of Style*, *JAMA*, *Scientific Style and Format*, and *Pediatrics* magazine are among the publications now using the non-possessive form. MedStudy will use the non-possessive form in these Q&A books when the proper name is followed by a common noun. So you will see phrasing such as "This patient would warrant workup for Crohn disease." Possessive form will be used, however, when an entity is referred to solely by its proper name without a following common noun. An example of this would be "The symptoms are classic for Crohn's."

MEDSTUDY
P. O. Box 38148
Colorado Springs, CO 80937
(800) 841-0547

ADOLESCENCE

1.

An 18-year-old female complains that her acne has continued to worsen since beginning an oral contraceptive several months earlier. She would prefer not to discontinue the oral contraceptive but is distraught about the appearance of her face. She reports no other side effects associated with oral contraceptive use.

Which of the following recommendations is most appropriate for this patient?

A. Change to another oral contraceptive with a higher estrogenic and lower androgenic effect.
B. Change to a progestin/estrogen vaginal ring.
C. Make no change in the type of oral contraceptive but begin oral antibiotic and topical therapy for acne.
D. Change to another oral contraceptive with a lower estrogenic and higher androgenic effect.
E. Change to a transdermal contraceptive patch.

2.

A 15-year-old male presents to the Emergency Room after being awakened by severe left testicular pain. He reports no history of preceding trauma and denies dysuria, frequency, or urethral discharge.

Which of the following findings is likely to be present if this patient's testicular pain is the result of torsion of the left testicle?

A. A brisk cremasteric reflex
B. Intense scrotal redness
C. A high riding testicle that lies on a horizontal plane
D. Relief of pain upon elevation of the testicle
E. A prominent tender bluish discoloration on the upper pole of the testicle

3.

A 17-year-old high school senior presents for a scheduled physical exam prior to college entry. She has been awarded an athletic scholarship for cross country and runs 50–60 miles/week. She has no complaints but does state that she hasn't had a menstrual period in 4 months. However, she enjoys not having to "hassle with it." She denies fasting, use of diuretics, emetics, or laxatives to control her weight and simply states that she "watches what she eats to be sure it's healthy." Her weight is in the 10th percentile and height in the 60th percentile. Her physical exam is remarkable only for a resting heart rate of 52. A pregnancy test is negative.

Which of the following recommendations is most appropriate for this patient?

A. Her daily intake of carbohydrates should increase by 50%.
B. An MRI of the head should be obtained to rule out a pituitary tumor.
C. Calcium and vitamin D supplementation should be prescribed.
D. She should be restricted from participating in competitive sports until her heart rate can be consistently documented to be ≥ 60 beats/minute.
E. An echocardiogram should be obtained to evaluate for evidence of ipecac induced cardiomyopathy.

4.

The parents of a 16-year-old male present with multiple concerns about the behavior of their son. They are fearful that he is "using drugs." They describe him as apathetic and uninterested in school and other extracurricular activities he once enjoyed. Although often lethargic with little to no apparent energy, he becomes easily frustrated and angry, often lashing out at his parents over "minuscule things like being asked to take out the trash." His academic performance has declined as has his overall appearance and dress. He has several "new friends" whom he refuses to introduce to his parents.

Which of the following substances is most likely to be detected on a urine drug screen in this patient?

    A. Tetrahydrocannabinol
    B. Cocaine
    C. Methamphetamine
    D. Methylamphetamine (MDMA)
    E. Lysergic acid diethylamide (LSD)

5.

A 16-year-old female presents with her parents who express concern about their daughter's weight loss. Reportedly she "eats next to nothing most of the time" and has lost nearly 30 pounds over a 6-month period of time. She appears angry and withdrawn, wearing multiple layers of baggy clothes. Her heart rate is 52 beats/minute, and blood pressure is 90/65.

Which of the following clinical findings is most suggestive that her weight loss is due, in part, to purging behaviors?

    A. Facial lanugo hair
    B. Yellowish-orange discoloration of the palms
    C. A systolic murmur associated with a mid-systolic click
    D. Parotid gland enlargement
    E. Acrocyanosis associated with dependent edema

6.

A sexually active 17-year-old female presents with the complaint of vaginal discharge for a period of several days. She states that the discharge is malodorous but denies associated pruritus, pain, or other additional symptoms. Her last menstrual period was 2 weeks ago. She uses an oral contraceptive but is on no other medications. On physical exam, a thin homogenous grayish white discharge is noted on the perineum. On saline wet prep numerous epithelial cells are noted to have a stippled cell membrane. Urine pregnancy test is negative.

Which of the following regimes represents the most appropriate treatment in this patient?

    A. Ceftriaxone 125 mg IM in a single dose
    B. Azithromycin 1g PO in a single dose
    C. Doxycycline 100 mg PO twice daily for 10 days
    D. Valacyclovir 1g PO twice daily for 7 days
    E. Metronidazole 500 mg PO twice daily for 7 days

7.

A 17-year-old female is transported to the Emergency Room after being found unresponsive and lying on the kitchen floor by her sister. She has a history of an eating disorder and has recently relapsed following a brief period of time where she was able to improve her diet and avoid self-induced vomiting. In the ER she is alert and states that "she just passed out for a second." During evaluation, an ECG is noted to have evidence of depression of the ST segments, flattened T waves and prominent U waves.

Which of the following laboratory findings is most likely to be the cause of the ECG findings?

    A. Serum creatinine of 2.1 mg/dL
    B. Serum potassium of 2.6 mmol/L
    C. Total serum calcium of 12.2 mg/dL
    D. Serum magnesium of 1.1 mg/dL
    E. Serum sodium of 128 mmol/L

8.

A 16-year-old male presents for a scheduled preparticipation sports physical prior to beginning football practice for his high school team. He states that he has "been lifting all summer" and hopes to win a starting spot on the team. He also shares that he has recently increased his caloric intake and has gained 25 pounds over the last 9 months. His blood pressure is 148/98. Height and weight are in the 85th percentile. An increase in muscle mass is noted when compared to his last visit. Abdominal striae are also present.

Which of the following complications is most likely to be associated with the illegal use of anabolic steroids in this patient?

    A. Acute pancreatitis
    B. Acute renal failure
    C. Myocardial infarction
    D. Cerebral vascular accident
    E. Drug induced hepatitis

9.

During a scheduled health maintenance exam, the mother of a 10-year-old boy inquires about pubertal changes that she should expect to occur in her son during the next several years.

Which of the following most accurately describes expected pubertal growth parameters in boys?

    A. Peak weight velocity follows peak height velocity by 9–12 months.
    B. Adult height can be predicted by adding 5 cm to the mother's height.
    C. During puberty the percentage of lean body mass decreases proportionately to an increase in the percentage of body fat.
    D. At the completion of puberty, testicular volume averages 20 mL.
    E. Peak height velocity occurs during sexual maturity rating (Tanner Stage) 2.

10.

During a scheduled well-child examination, the parents of 10-year-old twins—a boy and a girl—inquire about the onset of pubertal changes in their children.

Which of the following most accurately describes expected pubertal growth parameters?

A. The time of **onset** of increased growth velocity is similar in both boys and girls.
B. The **peak** height velocity occurs at a mean of 11.5 years in girls.
C. The **peak** height velocity occurs at a mean of 12.0 years in boys.
D. Pubertal growth accounts for about 10–15% of final adult height.
E. Growth during the year of **peak** height velocity averages 6.5 cm/year in girls.

11.

During a scheduled routine health-maintenance examination, a 13-year-old boy expresses concern that his peers have all "started to change" while he feels that he still "looks like a little kid."

Which of the following most accurately describes criteria for delayed puberty in males?

A. Genital Stage 1 persists beyond age 13.7 years.
B. Genital Stage 1 persists beyond 12.5 years.
C. Pubic Hair Stage 1 persists beyond 14.0 years.
D. More than 3 years have elapsed from initiation to completion of genital growth.
E. Genital Stage 2 persists for more than 1 year.

12.

The parents of a 16-year-old male present with concerns about their son's drug use. They describe him "as living only for his daily high." Once an honor student, he now frequently skips school or leaves early. He was recently arrested for shoplifting after he stole several CDs from a record store in the hope of selling them to obtain money to purchase drugs.

This patient's behavior is most consistent with which one of the following stages of adolescent drug use?

A. Stage 0
B. Stage 1
C. Stage 2
D. Stage 3
E. Stage 4

13.

A 15-year-old male is transported to the Emergency Room after his friends found him "acting weird." He is a known substance abuser who has had several previous drug-related visits to the ER since the recent divorce of his parents.

Which of the following findings is most consistent with inhalant abuse?

A. Lacrimation and rhinorrhea
B. Dry mouth and diaphoresis
C. Hypotonia and pinpoint pupils
D. Pneumothorax and pneumomediastinum
E. Nystagmus and decreased reflexes

14.

A 17-year-old female is transported to the Emergency Room after her friends found her in a hotel room crying hysterically that she "might have been raped." Earlier in the evening the patient and several friends attended a "hotel party" after a school dance. On physical examination there is evidence of vaginal bleeding and several vaginal lacerations. The patient has no recollection of the events of the evening soon after arriving at the hotel. There is concern that she may have inadvertently ingested a drug.

Which of the following substances is most likely to have been mixed with a drink unbeknownst to the victim?

A. Methaqualone
B. Nembutal
C. Rohypnol
D. Alprazolam
E. Chlorpromazine

15.

A 16-year-old girl presents to the Emergency Room after the principal at her school noted her to be "acting like she was high again." The principal plans to inform the girl's parents that she will not be allowed back into school until she obtains treatment for substance abuse. She is suspected to chronically abuse barbiturates.

Assuming that she ingested a barbiturate within several hours prior to presentation to the ER, which of the following eye findings is most likely to be identified upon further evaluation of this patient?

A. Injection of the conjunctiva
B. Papilledema
C. Dilated pupils
D. Lateral nystagmus
E. Horizontal and/or vertical nystagmus

16.

A 14-year-old girl presents with concerns about the appearance of her skin. She has used several over-the-counter acne preparations to no avail and is becoming increasingly self conscious.

Which of the following most accurately describes the cause(s) of acne in the adolescent population?

   A. Increased levels of androgens weaken the walls of the pilosebaceous unit, leading to rupture of the follicular epithelium.
   B. Excessive sebum production provides an ideal growth medium for excessive proliferation of *Staphylococcus aureus*.
   C. Oxidation leads to discoloration and darkening of closed comedones.
   D. The pilosebaceous follicles become plugged by androgen-induced proliferation of squamous cells within the lining of the follicle.
   E. Bacteria within the pilosebaceous follicle release chemotactic factors that attract neutrophils, which release lysosomal enzymes leading to inflammatory changes.

17.

A 19-year-old female wishes to begin oral contraceptives.

Which one of the following medications, when co-administered with an oral contraceptive, is most conclusively associated with interference with contraceptive effectiveness?

   A. Trimethoprim-sulfamethoxazole
   B. Fluoxetine
   C. Ciprofloxacin
   D. Hydrochlorothiazide
   E. Carbamazepine

18.

After hearing many players discuss the perceived benefits of creatine, several high school coaches request additional information about creatine use in young athletes.

Which of the following sports is most likely associated with the use of creatine among its players?

   A. Tennis
   B. Volleyball
   C. Wrestling
   D. Basketball
   E. Swimming

19.

During a scheduled health supervision visit, the mother of a 10-year-old girl questions when she can expect her daughter's "growth spurt" to occur.

During which of the following is the peak height velocity most likely to occur in girls?

A. Tanner stage 1–2
B. Tanner stage 2–3
C. Tanner stage 3–4
D. Tanner stage 4–5
E. The 3–6 months prior to onset of menses

20.

During a scheduled health supervision visit, the mother of a 10-year-old boy questions when she can expect her son to begin puberty.

Which of the following is the first to occur during pubertal development in males?

A. Sparse straight pubic hair along the base of the penis
B. Increase in the length of the penis
C. Darkening of the scrotal sac
D. Deepening of the voice
E. Increase in testicular volume

21.

A 17-year-old female's parents are convinced that she has "the mumps." The girl also complains of a sore throat and fatigue. On physical examination bilateral parotid gland enlargement is noted. Scattered soft palate petechiae are present on examination of the oropharynx, without associated tonsillar exudate or enlargement. Dental hygiene appears poor.

Which of the following laboratory results is most likely to be identified during additional evaluation of this patient?

A. Potassium: 5.1 mEq/L
B. Bicarbonate: 18 mEq/L
C. Chloride: 111 mEq/L
D. Potassium: 2.4 mEq/L
E. Sodium: 151 mEq/L

22.

A 16-year-old male presents with a history of poor school performance, irritability, and oppositional behavior at home. His parents are concerned that he is abusing drugs. On physical examination, prominent conjunctival irritation is noted.

Which of the following substances is a common cause of this physical finding?

A. Cocaine
B. Marijuana
C. Amphetamines
D. Alcohol
E. MDMA (3,4 methylenedioxymethamphetamine)

23.

A 16-year-old female with a history of anorexia nervosa has been "forcing herself to eat all she can and more" over the previous 2 weeks in an attempt to avoid hospitalization and "prove to her parents that she is not sick." Upon presentation, she is irritable and at times appears confused. Vital signs include a heart rate of 130 and a respiratory rate of 36. A gallop rhythm is noted on cardiac exam, as is lower extremity edema.

Which of the following laboratory findings is likely to be identified during additional evaluation of this patient?

A. Hypophosphatemia
B. Hypochloremia
C. Hypermagnesemia
D. Hyperkalemia
E. Hypernatremia

24.

A 15-year-old male presents with a 4-hour history of severe left testicular pain. There is no history of preceding trauma, dysuria, frequency, or urethral discharge. He denies sexual activity. Testicular torsion is suspected.

Which of the following describes a historical or clinical finding consistent with the diagnosis of testicular torsion?

A. The affected testis is characteristically tender to palpation but is rarely swollen.
B. The affected side is often lower than the contralateral side.
C. Prior episodes of testicular pain are unusual.
D. Elevation of the scrotum on the affected side results in relief of pain.
E. The cremasteric reflex is usually absent.

ALLERGY / IMMUNOLOGY / RHEUMATOLOGY

25.

In an 18-month-old who has had 4 episodes of wheezing, which of the following is <u>not</u> a risk factor for continued wheezing at age 6?

A. Anaphylactic reaction to peanuts
B. Never breastfed
C. Atopic dermatitis
D. Maternal asthma

26.

A 12-month-old has had atopic dermatitis requiring daily therapy for 6 months.

Compared to the general population of infants, which of the following is he more likely to have at age 12?

A. Contact dermatitis
B. Pityriasis rosea
C. Asthma
D. Cutaneous lymphoma

27.

A 4-year-old has had 3 episodes of lobar pneumonia. She has a fever today and WBC is 19,000 with 70% neutrophils. The lab calls to say the neutrophils are abnormal with very large inclusion bodies in the cytoplasm.

Which of the following is the most likely diagnosis?

A. Chronic granulomatous disease
B. Wiskott-Aldrich syndrome
C. Leukocyte adhesion deficiency
D. Chediak-Higashi disease

28.

Which of the following consists of the triad of thrombocytopenia, eczema, and immunodeficiency?

A. Chronic granulomatous disease
B. Ataxia-telangiectasia
C. Wiskott-Aldrich syndrome
D. Leukocyte adhesion deficiency

29.

Which of the following is characterized by a triad of DNA sensitivity to x-rays, cerebellar dysfunction, and immunodeficiency?

A. Chronic granulomatous disease
B. Ataxia-telangiectasia
C. Wiskott-Aldrich syndrome
D. Leukocyte adhesion deficiency

30.

Which of the following describes the triad of poor-to-absent healing of skin wounds, extreme neutrophilia, and early-onset periodontal disease?

A. Chronic granulomatous disease
B. Ataxia-telangiectasia
C. Wiskott-Aldrich syndrome
D. Leukocyte adhesion deficiency

31.

Which of the following describes a syndrome presenting with tissue-invasive infection (lymphadenitis, pneumonia, or abscess) with microorganisms of very low virulence?

A. Chronic granulomatous disease
B. Ataxia-telangiectasia
C. Wiskott-Aldrich syndrome
D. Leukocyte adhesion deficiency

32.

Which of the following is the most common trigger of asthma exacerbations in 10-year-olds?

A. Viral URI
B. Dust mite allergen
C. *Chlamydia* infection
D. Cat allergen

33.

A 5-year-old has had immediate allergic reactions to peanuts.

Which of the following is the approximate probability that she will react to another sort of nut?

  A. 5%
  B. 33%
  C. 67%
  D. 95%

34.

A 12-year-old boy is seen because he has had oral thrush most of the last 3 years and often before then. He also had esophageal candidiasis on endoscopy for complaint of heartburn. He has not had invasive bacterial infection or other opportunistic infection. On exam there are normal tonsils and lymph nodes without lymphadenopathy or hepatosplenomegaly. HIV-1 antibody testing is negative.

Which of the following is the most likely diagnosis?

  A. Severe combined immunodeficiency
  B. Wiskott-Aldrich syndrome
  C. HIV-2 infection
  D. Chronic mucocutaneous candidiasis

35.

A 14-year-old girl presents with complaints of low back pain that has gradually increased in intensity over the last 4–6 weeks. She does not have a history of associated trauma, although she participates in gymnastics most every afternoon after school. There is no history of associated fever or other systemic symptoms. On physical examination she has moderate point tenderness over the lower lumbar region that worsens when she's asked to bend backwards. There is also evidence of moderate hamstring tightness. Examination of the spine reveals no evidence of scoliosis, kyphosis, or lordosis.

Which one of the following is most likely to be identified upon further evaluation of this patient?

  A. Radiographic evidence of vertebral collapse associated with findings of acute lymphoblastic leukemia on bone marrow examination
  B. Spinal cord tumor on MRI
  C. Stress fracture of the pars interarticularis on bone scan
  D. Disc space narrowing and irregularities of the lower lumbar vertebral bodies on plain radiograph
  E. Marked forward slippage of L5 on S1 on lateral radiograph

36.

A 6-year-old boy presents with a 1-week history of intermittent abdominal pain, bilateral knee and left ankle pain. There are no associated systemic symptoms with the exception of two episodes of vomiting. On physical examination, periarticular swelling, tenderness, and decreased range of motion of both knees is noted. There is no associated warmth, erythema or effusion. The patient is treated symptomatically and instructed to return the following day for further laboratory evaluation. Upon return, his mother states that he has developed a new rash. On physical exam, there are scattered palpable purpuric lesions on the lower extremities along with several urticarial lesions around the ankles.

Which one of the following represents the most common cause of long-term morbidity in patients with this disorder?

    A. Chronic renal disease
    B. Progressive cardiomyopathy
    C. Severe debilitating arthritis
    D. Chronic persistent hepatitis
    E. Chronic pancreatitis

37.

An 11-year-old boy presents with pain in his left heel and foot. He has reproducible pain in his lower back as well. You order an ESR, and it returns at 9. An HLA-B27 test returns positive. His father had similar symptoms as a teenager and continues into adulthood.

Which of the following is most likely?

    A. JRA
    B. Juvenile psoriatic arthritis
    C. Lyme disease
    D. Gonococcal disease
    E. Spondyloarthropathy

38.

Which of the following findings increases the risk of having uveitis in a patient with oligoarticular JRA?

    A. Increased ESR
    B. Positive ANA
    C. Positive ds-DNA
    D. Positive erosions on hand x-rays
    E. Positive RF

39.

A 12-year-old girl presents with arthritis of her left knee and hand. On physical exam you note dactylitis and pitting of her nails. The DIP joints of her hand are most severely affected by the arthritis. An ANA returns and is positive.

Which of the following is most likely?

   A. JRA
   B. Spondyloarthropathy
   C. Juvenile psoriatic arthritis
   D. SLE
   E. Mixed connective tissue disease

40.

Which of the following is the correct treatment of Lyme meningitis?

   A. Oral doxycycline
   B. Ceftriaxone
   C. Vancomycin
   D. Ceftriaxone and vancomycin
   E. IV doxycycline

41.

A 12-year-old girl presents with chorea-like movements, which she cannot seem to control. At first her mother thought she was just "fooling around," but then the mother realized that she could not control them. She has no history of sore throat. She has oral ulcers and the following laboratory abnormalities: proteinuria, anemia and leukopenia, and pleuritis on CXR. ASO titer is 1:40.

Which of the following is the most likely diagnosis?

   A. Rheumatic fever
   B. Systemic lupus erythematosus (SLE)
   C. Juvenile rheumatoid arthritis (JRA)
   D. Behçet disease
   E. Post-streptococcal disease

42.

A 12-year-old-girl presents with severe urticaria, facial flushing, and tongue swelling after a bee sting. Her sister had a similar reaction to contrast dye.

Which of the following describes how a bee sting causes anaphylaxis?

    A. By causing an IgE mediated event against protein-hapten conjugants.
    B. By causing a direct activation of mediator release from mast cells, basophils, or both.
    C. By causing an IgE mediated reaction against the proteins in the sting media.
    D. It's a result of a deficiency of C1 esterase inhibitor.
    E. By causing an IgA mediated reaction against protein-hapten conjugants.

43.

An 8-year-old girl with no prior medical history presents for evaluation of a sore throat. Her eldest sister has a history of anaphylaxis to contrast dye, and her other older sister has a history of anaphylaxis to bee stings. You are able to confirm *Streptococcus pyogenes*, and you start her on the appropriate oral antibiotic for this infection. She returns that afternoon to the Emergency Room with a complaint of urticaria and facial flushing, and her tongue starts to swell. She responds to therapy and is observed in the ER.

Which of the following describes the mechanism for her anaphylaxis?

    A. She had IgE recognition of protein-hapten conjugants.
    B. She had IgE recognition of native proteins.
    C. She had direct activation of mediator release from mast cells, basophils, or both.
    D. She has a deficiency of C1 esterase inhibitor.
    E. She somehow got exposed to contrast material while in your office.

44.

A 13-year-old girl presents with facial pain and nasal congestion. She reports she had the onset of sore throat and rhinorrhea 5 days ago. Over the past 48 hours she has had facial pressure over the maxillary sinus and green nasal discharge. On exam, T 99.2°, BP 110/70. Nose: swollen turbinates. Neck: no adenopathy. Chest examination is clear.

Which of the following would you recommend?

    A. Decongestants/nasal irrigation + amoxicillin
    B. Decongestants/nasal irrigation + TMP/sulfa
    C. Decongestants/nasal irrigation + amoxicillin/clavulanate
    D. Decongestants/nasal irrigation
    E. Decongestants/nasal irrigation + metronidazole

45.

An 8-year-old boy has an anaphylactoid reaction to contrast dye. He is well now.

Each of the following statements concerning <u>anaphylactoid</u> reactions is true <u>except</u>:

- A. They are usually immune responses.
- B. Examples include reaction to radiocontrast agents.
- C. They are not immunoglobulin E-dependent (IgE).
- D. They are systemic reactions.
- E. They have the same symptoms as anaphylaxis.

46.

A 16-year-old girl presents to the Emergency Room immediately after receiving a bee sting. She has a past history of anaphylaxis and had lost her emergent home epinephrine device.

She has urticaria but is not having hypotension.

Which of the following is indicated?

- A. Give aqueous epinephrine 0.5 mg IV.
- B. Give aqueous epinephrine 0.5 mg IM.
- C. Give IV methylprednisolone 2 mg/kg IV.
- D. Start a beta-blocker.
- E. Give aqueous epinephrine 0.5 mg SQ.

47.

A 17-year-old female presents to the Emergency Room with complaints of malaise, fever, chills, and "aching joints." On physical examination her temperature is 100.9° F. Her wrists and hands are not swollen but are clearly painful on range-of-motion testing. Scattered about her palms and fingers are several painful 2–4 mm necrotic appearing lesions. There are also several petechial and pustular lesions present on the distal portion of the right forearm. Additional clinical findings include pain, warmth, and erythema over the right shoulder without associated effusion.

Which one of the following findings is most likely to be identified upon further examination of this patient's skin lesions?

- A. Gram-negative intracellular diplococci
- B. Multinucleated giant cells
- C. Gram-positive diplococci in chains
- D. Budding yeast and pseudohyphae
- E. Gram-negative cocci and coccobacilli

48.

During an evaluation for a suspected immunodeficiency, a 7-year-old girl with a history of recurrent sinusitis and otitis media is found to have very low levels of serum IgA. Serum levels of IgG and IgM are normal.

For which of the following organisms is this patient at highest risk of infection?

    A. *Giardia lamblia*
    B. *Salmonella typhi*
    C. *Shigella flexneri*
    D. *Shiga*-toxin producing *Escherichia coli*
    E. *Campylobacter jejuni*

49.

A patient presents in referral for evaluation of arthritis thought to be due to Juvenile Rheumatoid Arthritis (JRA).

Which of the following patients is at highest risk of developing iridocyclitis?

    A. A 7-year-old boy with a history of fever, rash, arthritis in multiple large and small joints, pleuritis, pericarditis, and liver enzyme elevation
    B. A 15-year-old girl with a history of arthritis in multiple large and small joints and a positive rheumatoid factor (RF) and antinuclear antibody (ANA) in the absence of prominent systemic symptoms
    C. A 6-year-old girl with a history of arthritis in multiple large and small joints and a negative RF in the absence of prominent systemic symptoms
    D. A 12-year-old boy with evidence of arthritis in the sacroiliac joints and hips with a negative ANA and RF in the absence of prominent systemic symptoms
    E. A 4-year-old girl with evidence of arthritis in the left knee, right elbow, and both ankles with a negative RF and a positive ANA

50.

Which of the following can occur after the <u>initial</u> exposure to a foreign substance and does not require "prior" exposure?

    A. IgE-mediated respiratory allergic symptoms
    B. Serum sickness
    C. Immediate allergic reactions to stings of insects
    D. Delayed hypersensitivity reaction to tuberculin
    E. Food allergy

51.

A mother brings her 9-year-old daughter, Hanna, to see you for a fever that has lasted about 5–6 days. The mother is concerned that Hanna may have strep throat because the glands in her neck are swollen, and strep has been going around school. The mother has noticed that Hanna's hands have seemed a little swollen, and she has a rash. No runny nose, vomiting, or diarrhea, but she has had some abdominal pain. She seems to be getting worse.

PAST MEDICAL HISTORY: She has been very healthy except for multiple ear infections as an infant.
ALLERGIES: Penicillin
IMMUNIZATIONS: UTD
MEDICATIONS: Ibuprofen
FAMILY HISTORY: Brother has asthma, otherwise negative

PHYSICAL EXAMINATION:
T 102.5°   HR 110   BP 90/65   RR 30
General: ill-appearing and lethargic

HEENT:	Red conjunctiva
	TMs clear
Nose:	Slight congestion
	Oral pharynx: lips red and cracking
Neck:	Tender 3 cm right anterior cervical node
Heart:	Increased rate, regular rhythm with flow murmur
Lungs:	CTA bilaterally
Abd:	Slightly tender all over; liver down 2 cm below costal margin
Ext:	Pulses 2+
Skin:	Red maculopapular rash in inguinal area and on trunk

LABORATORY:

WBC:	17,000/mm^3 with 65% segs, 8% bands, 25% lymphs, 2% monos
Hgb:	11 mg/dL
Hct:	33%
MCV:	85
Platelets:	375,000
ESR:	30 mm/hr

Rapid strep:	Negative
ASO:	Negative
Monospot:	Negative
EBV titers:	Pending
U/A:	+leukocytes, no bacteria, all else negative
Blood cultures:	Pending

After you initiate appropriate drug therapy for this child, which of the following would be the most important person to consult?

A. Ophthalmologist
B. Rheumatologist
C. Nephrologist
D. Cardiologist
E. Neurologist

52.

You are seeing a 15-month-old girl who received her 1st MMR 6 days ago. Today she is seen and diagnosed with Kawasaki disease. She will receive her IVIG tonight.

Which of the following should you do about her recent MMR vaccination?

A. She will not need a repeat dose until she is 4–6 years of age.
B. She will need a repeat dose now.
C. She will need a repeat dose in 5 months.
D. She will need a repeat dose given 11 months after her IVIG.
E. Check her measles titer in 2 weeks; if adequate she does not need any further immunization until age 4–6 years.

53.

IVIG may be beneficial for all of the following conditions <u>except</u>:

A. IgA deficiency
B. Some children with pediatric HIV
C. Kawasaki disease
D. Common variable immunodeficiency
E. Severe combined immunodeficiency

54.

Okay, some immunology questions you just have to deal with. The Boards like to ask these, and there are really no patient scenarios to embellish them with. I could make it cute and sweet, but that wouldn't really ease your pain. You know that you hate these questions. So for the immunology sections, just know that you will get a lot of short torture questions that you are expected to know. Here is one of those now.

Which of the following is expressed the earliest during B-cell development?

A. Surface immunoglobulin M
B. Surface immunoglobulin G
C. Surface immunoglobulin E
D. Surface immunoglobulin A
E. Cytoplasmic μ chains

55.

A 17-year-old adolescent presents with episodes of abdominal pain and stress-induced edema of the lips and tongue. Occasionally with severe stress, he will have laryngeal edema also. His examination in between these episodes is completely normal.

He is likely to have a low functional or absolute level of which of the following?

A. C5A
B. C1 esterase inhibitor
C. IgE
D. Surface immunoglobulin A
E. Cyclooxygenase

56.

A 12-year-old girl presents with a history of recurrent fevers and associated sputum production. The sputum is fairly foul in its appearance and its smell. She has a past medical history of recurrent upper respiratory infections. Additionally, she has had *Giardia* diarrheal infection twice in the last 8 years.

Pertinent findings on her physical examination:
    Coarse crackles in the left chest with decreased air movement; positive for foul-smelling sputum
    She has an enlarged spleen with a span of 10 cm
LABORATORY:
    CBC is normal
    Serum IgG is 80 mg/dL (normal 800–1,500 mg/dL)
    Serum IgA is 20 mg/dL (normal 90–325 mg/dL)

Which of the following is the most appropriate treatment?

A. Monthly intravenous immunoglobulin
B. Corticosteroids
C. Splenectomy
D. Bone marrow transplantation
E. IgA transfusion

57.

A 6-year-old girl presents with recurrent sinopulmonary infections and has developed severe respiratory insufficiency. She has bronchiectasis on a chronic basis. Recently she has developed progressive cerebellar ataxia and oculocutaneous telangiectasia. She has depressed levels of IgA and IgE on laboratory testing. Additionally, she is noted to have anergy to cutaneous testing. She does not have adenosine deaminase deficiency.

Which of the following is her likely diagnosis?

A. Common variable immunodeficiency
B. An abnormality on chromosome 12
C. Severe combined immunodeficiency
D. Ataxia-telangiectasia syndrome
E. Cystic fibrosis

58.

A 16-year-old adolescent has had a 2-year history of recurrent rash. She describes the rash as "small bumps that itch." She describes them as reddish-brown in color. Additionally with these "bumps" she has had flushing of her face, dizziness, and some abdominal pain. If she "pushes" on the skin lesions, they actually itch more and become redder. She has noted that her attacks can occur after she drinks wine (at family weddings or celebrations) or if she takes an ibuprofen. She had an upper GI series done last week that showed an ulcer in her duodenum.

Which of the following is the most likely diagnosis?

A. Systemic mastocytosis
B. Common variable immunodeficiency
C. Anaphylaxis to several agents
D. Familial angioedema syndrome
E. Leukemia

59.

An 11-year-old boy presents with abdominal pain, nausea, and vomiting. With this episode he has noted a rash and complains of severe arthralgias. He has never had this before.

His physical examination is significant for palpable purpura on his buttocks and lower extremities. None of the lesions are above his waist. Additionally, he has guaiac-positive stool.

Laboratory is sent and is remarkable for a urinalysis that shows mild proteinuria and red blood cell casts. Other studies are normal, including his CBC.

Which of the following is the most likely diagnosis?

A. Leukemia
B. Anaphylaxis to a hapten
C. Anaphylaxis to a protein
D. Job syndrome
E. Henoch-Schönlein Purpura (HSP)

60.

Which of the following is true about T cells?

A. They lack readily detectable immunoglobulin of **any** class on their membranes.
B. They lack readily detectable immunoglobulin except for IgM on their membranes.
C. They lack readily detectable immunoglobulin except for IgA on their membranes.
D. They lack readily detectable immunoglobulin except for IgE on their membranes.
E. They lack readily detectable immunoglobulin except for IgD on their membranes.

61.

Which of the following is/are true about immunoglobulin A?

A. It is the predominant immunoglobulin in body secretions.
B. IgA exists as 2 subclasses.
C. IgA provides defense against local infections in the respiratory, gastrointestinal, and the genitourinary system.
D. IgA can prevent virus-binding to epithelial cells.
E. All of the statements are true.

62.

A 13-year-old with a history of recurrent sinopulmonary infections presents for evaluation. He recovers from these infections fairly quickly, but he has between 4 and 6 episodes a year. Recently he received an infusion of packed red blood cells after a major motor vehicle accident. During the infusion, he developed anaphylaxis. The blood bank and hospital checked for mismatch and found no evidence of incompatibility.

Which of the following is his likely underlying condition?

A. Terminal complement deficiency
B. Systemic mastocytosis
C. Isolated IgA deficiency
D. IgG deficiency
E. IgD deficiency

63.

Which of the following statements is/are true regarding immune-complex disease?

A. Immune complexes do not have to persist in the circulation for the development of renal manifestations.
B. Most immune complexes are removed by the reticuloendothelial system.
C. The rash of cutaneous necrotizing vasculitis is not an example of immune-complex disease.
D. Signs and symptoms of immune-complex disease develop from the deposition of immune complexes in the reticuloendothelial system.
E. All of the statements are correct.

64.

Class I HLA antigens are expressed on all cells except:

A. Mature red blood cells
B. Reticulocytes
C. Reticulocytes and mature red blood cells
D. White blood cells
E. Purkinje cells

65.

You are seeing a boy with Wiskott-Aldrich syndrome. He has recurrent eczema and bloody diarrhea.

Which of the following is true about his disease?

A. It is associated with low IgA.
B. It is associated with low IgE.
C. It is associated with low IgM.
D. He does not have increased susceptibility to infection.
E. It cannot be treated successfully with bone marrow transplantation.

66.

A 4-year-old child presents to the Emergency Room with a fever of 5 days to 103° F and severe sore throat. She appears toxic and complains of a generalized headache, myalgias, lethargy, and severe malaise. Her physical examination is remarkable for swollen, erythematous lips and tongue. She has cervical lymphadenopathy with one node measuring 2 x 3 cm. She has bilateral conjunctivitis, and her palms and soles are thickened, red, and swollen in appearance.

CBC is done and shows a WBC of 15,000 with a mild left shift; platelets are elevated at 550,000; she is not anemic. A rapid streptococcal antigen test is negative, and a Monospot is also negative.

Which of the following is the most likely diagnosis?

A. Cryoglobulinemia
B. Bacterial endocarditis
C. Toxic epidermal necrolysis
D. Kawasaki disease
E. Takayasu arteritis

67.

A 13-year-old African-American girl presents with profound weakness and minimal muscle pain. These symptoms began 2–3 weeks ago. Initially, she could no longer run up the stairs at school as she normally did. She is not short of breath nor does she have a cough. She denies any rashes or joint pain. Her energy levels have been dramatically reduced. She is having no problems with swallowing.

On examination, she is quite weak in her proximal muscle groups. She is barely able to rise from a seated position. Proximal muscles in the upper extremities are similarly weakened, but distal muscle strength is normal, and there are no sensory deficits detected. Vital signs are normal. The joints have a good range of motion and are without active synovitis. Cutaneous exam is positive both for heliotrope and Gottron plaques. The remainder of her examination is normal.

Lab findings reveal a hemoglobin of 11.3, WBC of 12.1, and normal platelet count. Creatinine is normal. Creatinine kinase is 19,512. A muscle biopsy reveals fairly non-specific lymphocytic and neutrophil infiltrates of some of the muscle fibers, with occasional areas of necrosis. An EMG shows insertional irritability, positive sharp waves, and bizarre high-frequency repetitive discharges.

Which of the following is her most likely diagnosis?

A. SLE
B. Scleroderma
C. JRA
D. Dermatomyositis
E. Muscular dystrophy

68.

A 12-year-old girl with newly diagnosed systemic lupus erythematosus presents for follow-up. She has been doing fairly well over the last 3 months.

Which of the following is associated with a <u>worse</u> prognosis?

A. Nephritis
B. Fever and leukocytosis
C. Rash
D. Seizures
E. Anti-DNA antibodies

69.

You are seeing a 13-year-old girl with a recent diagnosis of juvenile rheumatoid arthritis (JRA). She has multiple small and large joints affected by her arthritis. She has been diagnosed as having polyarticular JRA. Her rheumatoid factor (RF) is pending.

Which of the following is true regarding her disease?

A. If the RF is negative, she will likely have more aggressive disease.
B. If the RF is positive, she will likely have more aggressive disease.
C. She is likely to have a negative ANA if her RF is positive.
D. She is likely to have a negative ANA if her RF is negative.
E. If the RF is negative, this usually indicates an HLA association.

70.

An 18-year old student is referred to your office from campus health care. There is a concern that she has a possible connective tissue disease process. She lives in Florida at home during the summer months but attends school in the Northeast during the winter months. Over the last month or two of severe winter weather, she has noticed that her fingers seem to be quite painful and go through some color changes, which are brand new to her. Most specifically, her fingers are initially white and then seemingly go a little blue and then remain red for prolonged periods of time. She struggles to complete her projects because she finds it very difficult to type. She thinks her finger joints are a little painful. She readily admits to some alcohol intake and has recently begun to smoke 5–10 cigarettes per day, particularly more so over the weekends. She denies any rashes, shortness of breath, or cough. She has no problem swallowing food. As part of her workup on campus, she was found to have a strongly positive anti-nuclear antibody. She had been reading about lupus and was very concerned about this condition, particularly from the information that she had gleaned from the Internet.

On examination, she is alert and oriented. BP is 112/57, pulse is 76. All pulses are present and equal. She has no bruits. There is a negative Allen's test. Cardiorespiratory exam is benign. Musculoskeletal exam is benign. Cutaneous exam reveals no rashes, vasculitis, or pulp atrophy. There is a negative vital capillaroscopy. Lab findings include a positive ANA in a titer of 1:320, with normal being less than 1:40. Hemoglobin was 11.9, and WBC was 4.9. UA is negative.

Which of the following would further appropriate workup include?

    A. ECHO to estimate pulmonary pressure
    B. Bronchoscopy
    C. Repeat ANA, anti-ds-DNA titers, anti-centromere, and anti-SCL70
    D. Esophageal manometry
    E. Upper extremity arteriography

71.

A 14-year-old female is seen in the outpatient setting for painful and swollen knees and feet. These symptoms began about 10 days ago. She describes the pain as incapacitating, can barely ambulate, and is brought in today in a wheelchair. She has never had any joint pain prior to this. She denies any rashes. She thinks that she had a fever about 2 weeks ago. The fever developed 2–3 days into a weeklong trip to Mexico that she was on. Toward the end of that trip, she developed fairly significant diarrhea for about 48 hours, which was quickly self-limiting. No rectal bleeding was noted at that time. She has had no urinary symptoms since then.

On examination, her temperature was 97.3° F. She was not pale or jaundiced. BP was 112/72 and pulse was 100. Cardiac and respiratory exams were benign. Cutaneous exam was benign. Musculoskeletal exam revealed no upper extremity joint synovitis. However, she had very significant knee effusions. Also, she was very tender over the insertion of the right Achilles' tendon and had significant sausaging asymmetrically of several of the lower extremity digits.

Which of the following is the proper course of action?

    A. Admit the patient and place her on broad-spectrum IV antibiotics.
    B. Inject both knees with corticosteroids.
    C. X-ray both knees and ankles.
    D. Systemic corticosteroids.
    E. Check baseline labs to include CBC, Sed rate, RF, and aspirate one of the knees.

72.

Which of the following is <u>not</u> a major manifestation of the Jones Criteria for the diagnosis of rheumatic fever?

    A. Arthralgia
    B. Carditis
    C. Erythema marginatum
    D. Subcutaneous nodules
    E. Chorea

73.

Which of the following is <u>most</u> likely to occur as an <u>isolated</u> manifestation of rheumatic fever?

  A. Carditis
  B. Fever
  C. Chorea
  D. Erythema marginatum
  E. Subcutaneous nodules

74.

A 15-year-old female presents to your office with the complaint of bilateral knee pain and swelling that started the day before. She denies trauma. She states she has felt warm today. No vomiting or diarrhea. She does complain of some dysuria today. Also her eyes have been red and burning today. She was treated about 10 days ago for *Chlamydia*.

On physical examination, her temp is 100.9° F. Conjunctivae are red. She also has bilateral knee pain and swelling. She does have decreased range of motion of both knees due to the swelling. The rest of the exam is normal.

Urine dipstick shows 2+ leukocytes.

Which of the following is the most likely diagnosis?

  A. Spondyloarthropathy
  B. Reactive arthritis (Reiter syndrome)
  C. Ankylosing spondylitis
  D. Dermatomyositis
  E. Juvenile rheumatoid arthritis

75.

A 20-month-old male presents with fever, cough, and mild respiratory distress and is subsequently diagnosed with pneumonia. His history is positive for several additional episodes of pneumonia, as well as 2 occurrences of a perirectal abscess, despite appropriate antimicrobial therapy and surgical intervention. In addition to the respiratory symptoms, his current physical exam also reveals cervical and inguinal adenopathy. His brother and two male cousins also have a history of recurrent pneumonia and skin infections.

Which of the following studies is most likely to indicate the etiology of this patient's disorder?

  A. IgG, IgM, and IgA immunoglobulin levels
  B. Antibody levels to vaccine antigens—tetanus, diphtheria, and *H. influenzae*
  C. Platelet count
  D. *Candida* or tetanus toxoid skin tests
  E. Nitroblue tetrazolium (NBT) test

CARDIOLOGY

76.

Prostaglandin E1 (PGE1) is useful for the palliation in the neonate for which of the following?

A. Mitral regurgitation
B. Tricuspid regurgitation
C. Critical coarctation of the aorta
D. Total anomalous pulmonary venous return
E. Ventricular septal defect

77.

Left axis deviation on the electrocardiogram is seen in which of the following pair of conditions?

A. Ventricular septal defect; aortic stenosis
B. Aortic stenosis; patent ductus arteriosus
C. Pulmonary atresia; tricuspid atresia
D. Tricuspid atresia; ventricular septal defect
E. Tricuspid atresia; AV canal defect

78.

A 14-year-old female presents with chest pain x 3 days. The pain is constant and located over the mid-precordium. An ECG is obtained and shown below:

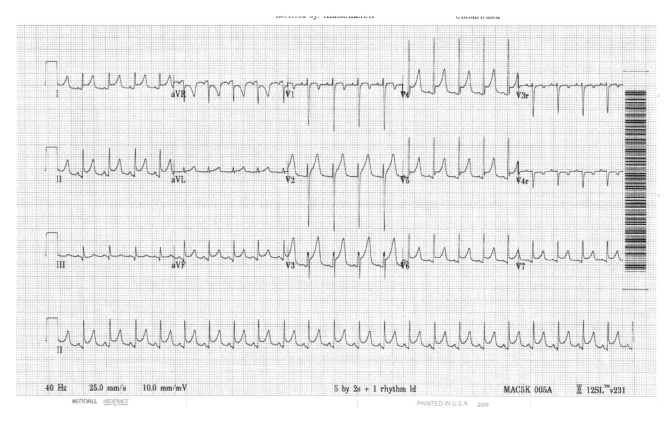

Based on this ECG, which of the following is the most likely etiology of her chest pain?

    A. Severe aortic stenosis
    B. Benign chest pain ("precordial catch syndrome")
    C. Pneumonia
    D. Mitral valve prolapse
    E. Pericarditis

79.

A 7-year-old female is referred to your office for a heart murmur. The ECG, obtained prior to your office visit, is shown below:

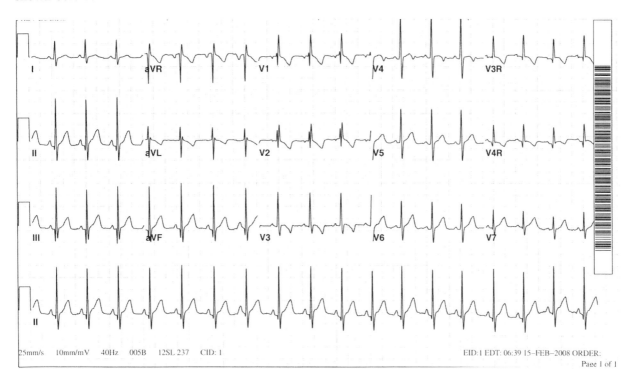

25mm/s   10mm/mV   40Hz   005B   12SL 237   CID: 1   EID:1 EDT: 06:39 15-FEB-2008 ORDER:

Page 1 of 1

Based on this ECG, which of the following is the most likely diagnosis?

A. VSD
B. PDA
C. ASD
D. Coarctation of the aorta
E. Innocent murmur

80.

A 16-year-old female has suffered from recurrent syncope for years. She has been relatively resistant to standard treatments for neurocardiogenic syncope (increasing fluids, mineralocorticoids, alpha-adrenergic agonists). She has had very extensive workups, including tilt tests, MRIs, complete metabolic panels, and thyroid function testing, all which have been normal. You obtain an ECG after she recovers from a fainting episode in your office:

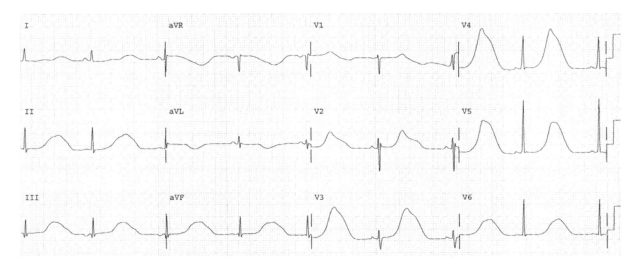

Based on this tracing, you should initiate therapy with which of the following?

    A. Digoxin
    B. High-dose aspirin
    C. Propranolol
    D. Glucose-insulin drip
    E. Fludrocortisone (Florinef®)

81.

A 4-day-old male, born at term to a 24-year-old woman, is noted to be cyanotic. His cardiac examination is positive for a displaced PMI, a gallop rhythm, and a holosystolic murmur that is especially prominent along the anterior left side of the chest. His chest x-ray shows prominent cardiomegaly. Review of the mother's chart indicates that her other two children were removed from her home due to medical neglect. She went into labor while hospitalized at an inpatient psychiatric facility after outpatient medical intervention proved unsuccessful.

Which of the following represents the most likely diagnosis in the infant's mother?

    A. Depression
    B. Schizophrenia
    C. Munchausen syndrome
    D. Crack cocaine addiction
    E. Bipolar disease

82.

During a preparticipation sports physical for basketball, a 16-year-old male is noted to have a mid-systolic click on cardiac exam. He wears glasses, is tall for his age, has a reduced upper segment-to-lower segment ratio, and has mild scoliosis.

In addition to mitral valve prolapse, which of the following is most likely to be identified during an echocardiogram in this patient?

A. Asymmetric septal hypertrophy
B. Atrial septal defect
C. Dilated aortic root
D. Bicuspid aortic valve
E. Dilated right atrium

83.

A previously well 16-year-old male is referred following a syncopal episode during a high school basketball game. His coach reports that the patient was alert "within seconds." There was no associated seizure activity. In addition, the patient's cousin suddenly died while jogging a year earlier. An echocardiogram is positive for marked hypertrophy of the interventricular septum.

Which of the following represents a commonly associated finding in patients with this disorder?

A. A systolic murmur heard best at the apex and left lower sternal border, which increases in intensity when moving from an upright to a supine position
B. A systolic murmur heard best at the left upper sternal border, which decreases in intensity with the Valsalva maneuver
C. A diastolic murmur heard best at the left upper sternal border while standing
D. A harsh murmur present during both systole and diastole heard best at the right and left second intercostal space
E. A midsystolic click heard best when sitting and leaning forward

84.

During a scheduled well-child examination, a 4-year-old boy is found to have a heart murmur. His parents report no concerns about his ability to exercise and keep up with peers. He takes no daily medications, has no known allergies, and has never been hospitalized. Blood pressure is 86/52 mmHg in the right arm; heart rate is regular at 66 beats/minute. The intensity of the murmur is II/VI and is heard best over the anterior portion of the upper chest during both systole and diastole. As the patient is asked to move his head up and down and side to side, the intensity of murmur is noted to vary with the position of the head. No extra heart sounds or rubs are identified. The pulses are equal and symmetric in the upper and lower extremities.

Which of the following is the most appropriate next step in the evaluation of this patient?

A. PA and lateral chest x-ray.
B. Electrocardiogram.
C. The parents can be assured that additional evaluation is not required.
D. Echocardiogram.
E. CT of the chest.

85.

An 18-year-old male presents for a college physical. He states that he has a "heart condition" and requests a prescription for antibiotics to have available "prior to any dental visit."

According to the American Heart Association recommendations, which of the following would require antimicrobial prophylaxis in this patient?

A. Bicuspid aortic valve
B. Mitral valve prolapse with regurgitation
C. Hypertrophic cardiomyopathy with resting obstruction
D. A prosthetic heart valve
E. Complete repair of a VSD at 4 years of age with a prosthetic material

86.

A 19-year-old man dies after dropping a 15-pound weight on his chest while exercising and lifting weights at a gym. He had no history of previous respiratory or cardiac disease and was considered to be in excellent physical condition. His friends report that he seemed to "pass out within seconds" after the accident and "never woke up" in spite of their attempts at resuscitation.

Which of the following is the most likely cause of death in this patient?

A. Tension pneumothorax
B. Pericardial tamponade
C. Respiratory arrest
D. Ventricular fibrillation
E. Coronary artery tear

87.

A 17-year-old boy with a history of a bicuspid aortic valve presents with fever and malaise associated with a "rash" first noticed the day prior to presentation. On physical examination, his temperature is 101.9° F. He appears fatigued. He is hospitalized and subsequently is found to have three separate blood cultures, which are positive for viridans streptococci.

Which of the following best describes expected findings on examination of this patient's skin and mucous membranes?

A. Desquamation of the hands and feet
B. Erythema and cracking of the lips
C. Macular, blanching painful lesions limited to the trunk
D. Painful, violaceous nodules in the pulp of the fingers and toes
E. Intensely erythematous fine maculopapular rash most prominent in the groin, axilla, and trunk

88.

A 17-year-old female is noted to be at the 95th percentile for height. Additional physical findings include arachnodactyly, scoliosis, and pectus excavatum. She also has a history of myopia. During her most recent visit to an ophthalmologist, she was diagnosed with subluxation of the crystalline lens of her right eye. Further evaluation for associated cardiac abnormalities is recommended.

Which of the following findings is most likely to be identified during echocardiography in this patient?

A. Ventricular septal defect
B. Enlarged right atrium associated with displaced septal and posterior leaflets of the tricuspid valve
C. Coarctation of the aorta
D. Dilation of the aortic root
E. Asymmetric hypertrophy of the interventricular septum

89.

You are seeing a 2-year-old for the first time for a well-child exam. The mother reports he has had a few ear infections but is otherwise very healthy. His immunizations are up to date, and he is developmentally normal. On physical examination, he is playful and active, and vital signs are normal. Everything appears fine, except you hear a systolic ejection murmur best heard at the left upper sternal border.

Which of the following would make you suspect an atrial septal defect (ASD)?

A. Fixed split second sound
B. Early systolic ejection click
C. Cyanosis
D. Midsystolic click
E. Greater arterial pulses in the upper extremities compared to the lower

90.

You are called to the nursery STAT following a normal term delivery of a female infant. The nurse reports that the infant looks blue. The mother had a normal pregnancy (without infection) and delivery. There has been no fever in either the mother or the infant. You arrive at the nursery to see a female infant with bluish discoloration of the skin and mucous membranes, which worsen with crying. You administer 100% oxygen for 10 minutes and get an arterial PO_2, which is 80 mmHg.

Which of the following would be your <u>immediate</u> course of action?

    A. Order a chest x-ray and ECG
    B. Order a cardiac catheterization
    C. Observation for 12 hours
    D. Start prostaglandin E1 following echocardiography diagnosis
    E. Intubate since this is caused by respiratory pathology

91.

You are called to see a 1-day-old in the nursery for an erratic heart rate. On the monitor, the HR ranges from 80 to 130. You obtain an ECG, which shows a corrected QT interval of 0.48 sec. The infant appears stable.

Which of the following would you recommend for this infant?

    A. Amiodarone
    B. Bretylium
    C. Radiofrequency ablation
    D. Propranolol
    E. No treatment is necessary

92.

Here is a straightforward knowledge question. Occasionally, they will throw this type of question at you.

Which of the following is the most common cyanotic heart defect <u>manifesting in newborns</u>?

    A. Tetralogy of Fallot
    B. Total anomalous pulmonary venous return
    C. Transposition of the great vessels
    D. Tricuspid atresia
    E. VSD

93.

A 2-year-old child comes into the emergency room with severe cyanosis. The parents say the child has a congenital heart defect. You note that the child is squatting when he is left alone.

PAST MEDICAL HISTORY: Negative except for knowledge of congenital heart defect

SOCIAL HISTORY: Attends daycare
Lives with mother and father; neither smoke

FAMILY HISTORY: Non-contributory
No siblings with congenital heart disease

REVIEW OF SYSTEMS: Decreased appetite recently

PHYSICAL EXAMINATION:
BP 80/40 (normal), P 120 (tachycardic), RR 30 (tachypneic), Temp 98.5° F
Cyanosis is evident
Heart: Relatively quiet sounds; right ventricular impulse is noted
Pulmonary closure is not heard

Rest of exam: okay

Well, let's make this easy for you. This is an older child with congenital heart disease and cyanosis. The most common etiology for this is tetralogy of Fallot. His physical examination and the noted squatting are consistent with this diagnosis.

Which of the following are the 4 components of tetralogy of Fallot?

    A. Large VSD, right ventricular outflow tract obstruction, overriding aorta, RVH
    B. Large VSD, left ventricular outflow tract obstruction, overriding aorta, LVH
    C. Large VSD, right ventricular outflow tract obstruction, overriding aorta, LVH
    D. ASD, VSD, patent ductus arteriosus, LVH
    E. ASD, right ventricular outflow tract obstruction, overriding aorta, RVH

94.

A 17-year-old female presents to your office complaining of palpitations. These occur most often when she drinks coffee. She has never had syncope. The palpitations can last up to 3–5 minutes and spontaneously resolve.

PAST MEDICAL HISTORY: Negative

SOCIAL HISTORY: Married with 1 child. Smokes 2 packs/day of cigarettes

FAMILY HISTORY: Mother 60 with HTN. Father 50 with HTN

REVIEW OF SYSTEMS: Negative

PHYSICAL EXAMINATION:
BP 110/70, P 90, RR 16, Temp 98.8°, Ht. 6'1", Wt 230 lbs

HEENT:	PERRLA, EOMI
	TMs clear
	Throat clear
Neck:	Supple
Heart:	RRR without murmurs, rubs, or gallops
Lungs:	CTA
Abdomen:	Benign
Extremities:	No cyanosis, clubbing, or edema
GU:	Normal female external genitalia

Which of the following would be the most useful test in evaluation of this patient?

A. Stress test
B. Left heart catheterization
C. Holter study
D. Right heart catheterization
E. Echocardiogram

95.

A local dentist calls wanting to know about endocarditis prophylaxis for his patients. He gives you a list of items he is concerned about and asks your opinion if they require prophylaxis.

Which of the following requires prophylaxis for dental procedures?

A. Isolated secundum atrial septal defect
B. Primum atrial septal defect
C. Presence of an implanted defibrillator with epicardial leads
D. Mitral valve prolapse with a significant audible murmur
E. None of the choices require antibiotic prophylaxis for dental procedures

---

96.

A dentist calls wanting to know about which dental procedures require prophylaxis, if clinically indicated. She gives you a list that she is concerned about.

Which of the following dental procedures requires prophylaxis for endocarditis?

A. Orthodontic appliance adjustment
B. Initial placement of orthodontic bands
C. Suture removal
D. Impressions
E. Placement of removable orthodontic appliances

97.

A 16-year-old high school student collapses at mid-court during a basketball game after a thunderous game-ending dunk shot. You assist in his full resuscitation from ventricular fibrillation, accompanied in this effort by the local paramedics who were there in 3½ minutes.

With an opportunity to examine him in the hospital, you are struck by his bifid carotid impulses, which are mirrored in his apex cardiogram, the latter of which you are able to both palpate and project via shadows on the bed clothing. He has a harsh holosystolic murmur at the lower left sternal border that accentuates with the upright posture, as well as with the Valsalva strain. Occasional premature contractions are followed by radial artery impulses, which are diminished relative to the apparent sinus cycle pulsations.

Which of the following is the most likely diagnosis?

    A. Myxomatous mitral valve prolapse (MVP)
    B. Hypertrophic obstructive cardiomyopathy (HOCM or IHSS)
    C. Ostium secundum atrial septal defect (ASD)
    D. Ostium primum atrioventricular septal defect (AVSD)
    E. Acquired (muscular) ventricular septal defect (VSD)

98.

You are on duty in the emergency room when a group of four companions bring in their friend, a 16-year-old female. She has scars from acute and chronic intravenous drug use. She is acutely ill with a temperature of 104° F, IIR 130/min, respirations 18/minute, and in apparent distress. Her systemic venous pressure is elevated, and the jugular venous pulse contour is dominated by large "cv" waves that swell with each inspiration. Your auscultatory examination reveals a Grade III/VI holosystolic murmur heard best at the lower left (and right) sternal border(s), and which accentuates to Grade IV/VI intensity with inspiration. The liver seems to pulsate with each systole.

A chest x-ray reveals scattered focal white fluffy opacities.

Which of the following is the most likely heart abnormality?

    A. Tricuspid regurgitation
    B. Mitral regurgitation
    C. Aortic valvular regurgitation
    D. Ruptured sinus of Valsalva aneurysm
    E. Bleeding pulmonary arteriovenous (AV) fistula

99.

You staff the outpatient clinic of your local hospital one afternoon when both parents present their 6-year-old son. They are concerned that he has not been able to start school. He has seemed to them to have "weak muscles," which have resulted in a "funny way of walking," as well as frequent falls and difficulty in arising from a chair or ascending the stairs at night at bedtime. They describe a curious method of arising from the floor wherein he "walks up" his torso (using a hands-to-knees sequence, which you recognize as Gower sign). On your examination, you are struck by the apparent hypertrophy of his calf muscles.

Which of the following is correct?

A. They may expect a normal life span for their son.
B. They must be aware of the risk of sudden death.
C. Happily, his children will have little or no chance of disease.
D. Sadly, should they decide to have additional children, all of his sisters theoretically could be similarly affected.
E. He is at risk for premature myocardial infarction.

100.

A 17-year-old high school student seeks a pre-employment physical from you prior to applying for the position of lifeguard at the Stone Mountain Country Club Pool. You note his tall, thin habitus and obtain height and arm-span measurements of 72" each. Your examination documents a Grade II/VI systolic ejection "flow" murmur in the pulmonary outflow tract and apparent fixed splitting of the second heart sound. His ECG demonstrates a mean electrical QRS avis of 115 degrees in the frontal plane, and there are prominent R waves in lead V_1 with an R:S ratio of (1.3:1).

You recognize that his apparent Type A right ventricular hypertrophy (RVH) is surely a result of which of the following?

A. Cystic fibrosis
B. Primary pulmonary hypertension
C. Ostium secundum atrial septal defect (ASD)
D. Membranous ventricular septal defect (VSD)
E. Wolff-Parkinson-White syndrome (WPW)

101.

A 16-year-old male collapses and dies during a sprint at a track meet. He was previously healthy and had no abnormalities on his school's routine physical examination for athletes.

Which of the following is the most likely finding at autopsy?

A. Large mitral valve leaflets with infiltration of myxomatous material on microscopic examination
B. An anomalous origin of the left anterior descending coronary artery from the right coronary cusp
C. Hypertrophic cardiomyopathy with a grossly thickened interventricular septum
D. Severe pulmonic stenosis
E. No abnormalities

102.

An actress plays the part of one of four sisters who lived in Boston during the civil war. In the movie, she takes some bread to some starving immigrant neighbors, one of whom has scarlet fever. In the movie, a few years later, she is dying of a cardiac-related illness.

If this had been a real case, which of the following would she be most likely to have on physical examination?

A. A soft S_1
B. A soft, decrescendo blowing murmur heard at the lower left sternal border in the sitting position
C. A midsystolic click followed by a systolic murmur heard at the left sternal border
D. A sound heard with the diaphragm at the apex shortly after S_2
E. A sound heard best with the bell at the apex after S_2

103.

Parents rush their 18-month-old daughter into the ER. They were at a nearby park when she collapsed, and they don't know what happened. On rapid assessment, she is unresponsive and pale.

Your immediate next step would be which of the following?

A. Open airway and check breathing
B. Start chest compressions
C. Give 20 mL/kg of normal saline IV
D. Give epinephrine
E. Intubate

104.

A 9-year-old female is in your office with the complaint of dizziness and chest discomfort that started abruptly at school about one hour ago. No fever, vomiting, or diarrhea. She has had no recent illnesses and has been very healthy.

On physical examination, she is anxious but stable. Heart rate is 190. She has good color and pulses.

You get an electrocardiogram that shows a consistent rate of 190 beats/min, absent P waves, and a narrow QRS complex. Vagal maneuvers have been unsuccessful.

Which of the following is the next step you should take?

A. Immediate synchronized cardioversion
B. Continue trying vagal maneuvers until the child's condition no longer permits
C. Give beta-blockers
D. Establish vascular access to administer adenosine
E. Give lidocaine

105.

Tetralogy of Fallot is a relatively common disorder on ABP Board Exams.

Which of the following is <u>not</u> a clinical feature or common complication of tetralogy of Fallot?

A. Brain abscess
B. Congestive heart failure
C. Poor growth
D. Anoxic spells
E. Cyanosis

106.

A 6-month-old infant is brought in by his parents. He has had a cold for a day or two and today, his mother noted that he was "breathing fast." Physical examination: Shows an uncomfortable-appearing child in mild distress. He is tachypneic with a respiratory rate of 50. You note, however, that his pulse is extremely rapid—too rapid to count easily. He is febrile to 101° F. An emergent ECG is done. It shows a very regular rate of 282 beats per minute. You are not sure if you can discern P waves. The QRS complexes appear normal.

Which of the following is the most likely etiology of his tachycardia?

A. Supraventricular tachycardia with underlying congenital heart disease
B. Supraventricular tachycardia without underlying congenital heart disease
C. Ventricular tachycardia
D. Ventricular fibrillation
E. Sinus tachycardia

107.

Which of the following are the most common organisms to cause bacterial endocarditis in children?

A. Viridans streptococci, *Enterococcus*, and *Staphylococcus aureus*
B. *Haemophilus influenzae*, and *Streptococcus pneumoniae*
C. *Streptococcus pyogenes* and *Enterococcus*
D. *Streptococcus pyogenes*, *Haemophilus influenzae*, and *Streptococcus pneumoniae*
E. Anaerobes

108.

Anthony Craig is a 2-month-old boy who is hospitalized emergently because of severe dyspnea and cyanosis. CXR shows minimal cardiomegaly and a diffuse reticular pattern in all lung fields.

Which of the following is the most likely diagnosis?

A. Transposition of the great vessels
B. Hypoplastic left heart
C. Tricuspid atresia
D. Tetralogy of Fallot
E. Total anomalous pulmonary venous return with obstruction of the veins

109.

An infant with severe cyanosis presents. For some cases, balloon atrial septostomy can be lifesaving.

For which of the following conditions would this be helpful?

A. A large VSD
B. Transposition of the great vessels
C. Anomalous pulmonary venous return
D. Truncus arteriosus
E. Tetralogy of Fallot

110.

Which of the following is a feared complication of a VSD if the VSD is allowed to persist too long?

A. Spontaneous closure of the defect
B. Development of pulmonary valvular insufficiency
C. Brain tumors
D. Eisenmenger syndrome
E. Aplastic anemia

111.

Match the following syndromes/clinical settings with the <u>most commonly</u> associated congenital heart defects:

A. Williams syndrome _____
B. Down syndrome _____
C. Maternal lithium ingestion _____
D. Maternal diabetes _____
E. Fetal alcohol syndrome _____
F. Noonan syndrome _____
G. Turner syndrome _____

1. Transposition of great vessels
2. VSD, ASD
3. Coarctation of the aorta
4. Valvular pulmonic stenosis
5. Mitral regurgitation
6. Supravalvular aortic stenosis
7. Septal hypertrophy
8. Complete AV canal (AV septal defect)
9. Hypoplastic left ventricle
10. Ebstein anomaly of the tricuspid valve

112.

A 3-year-old child presents for a new visit and routine examination. You hear a systolic heart murmur and ask his mother about this. She says that no one has told her about this before. An ECG shows the following: Normal sinus rhythm with a rate of 100; right axis deviation (105 degrees), tall R waves over the right precordial leads, and deep S waves over the left precordial leads. There also is an rsR pattern in V1.

Which of the following is the most likely diagnosis?

A. Atrial septal defect
B. Ventricular septal defect
C. Coarctation of the aorta
D. Hypothyroidism
E. Endocarditis

113.

A child has an ECG. It shows an Rs pattern over the right precordium.

For which of the following is this Rs pattern normal?

A. An ECG in a 2-month-old infant.
B. An ECG in a 12-year-old.
C. An ECG in both a 12-year-old and a 2-month-old.
D. This is never normal.
E. This is always normal.

114.

A child has an ECG. It shows inverted T waves in V_3R and V_1.

For which of the following is this ECG finding normal?

A. The ECG of a 2-month-old.
B. The ECG of a 12-year-old.
C. The ECG of both a 12-year-old and a 2-month-old.
D. This is never normal except in the first few days of life.
E. This is normal in adults only.

115.

Which of the following is the average blood pressure at 2 years of age?

A. 50/30 mmHg
B. 80/20 mmHg
C. 95/60 mmHg
D. 120/80 mmHg
E. 70/40 mmHg

116.

An 8-year-old girl presents to your clinic for a routine health supervision examination. She is new to your practice, and the mother tells you she has been healthy all of her life. You obtain the following history:

HOSPITALIZATIONS:	None
SURGERY:	Appendectomy at 6 years of age
MEDICATIONS:	Multivitamin
ALLERGIES:	Amoxicillin with rash
DIET:	Normal for age
FAMILY HISTORY:	Non-contributory
SOCIAL HISTORY:	Mom and dad are separated. Your patient and her mother just recently moved to town to live with the grandparents. She will be in the third grade and has been an A–B student.
REVIEW OF SYSTEMS:	Negative for 10 systems

PHYSICAL EXAMINATION:
Afebrile HR: 72/minute, RR: 20/minute, Wt: 22 kg (25%), Ht: 123 cm (25%)

HEENT:	Clear
Chest:	Clear to auscultation
Heart:	Regular rate and rhythm with a 2/6 systolic ejection murmur best heard at the second intercostal space on the left of the sternum. There is fixed splitting of the second heart sound.
Abdomen:	Soft with no hepatosplenomegaly
Genitalia:	Normal
Skin:	Normal
Neuro:	Non-focal examination

Because of the heart murmur, you obtain a chest x-ray and an ECG.

Chest x-ray: Cardiomegaly with enlargement of the right atrium, right ventricle, and pulmonary artery
ECG: Right axis deviation with right ventricular hypertrophy

Which of the following cardiac defects does she have?

A. Atrial septal defect
B. Ventricular septal defect
C. Pulmonary stenosis
D. Innocent murmur
E. Patent ductus arteriosus

117.

A 12-year-old boy is referred to your clinic because, on a sports physical, he was found to have a blood pressure of 150/100 mmHg. The physician told the parents that he would need to be worked up before he could play football. The mother is very concerned about getting him cleared as soon as possible so he can play, since he is the star of the team. She seems irritated that she had to find a physician to see her son.

HOSPITALIZATIONS:	None
ALLERGIES:	None
MEDICATIONS:	None
SURGERY:	None

FAMILY HISTORY: 4 siblings, all alive and well

SOCIAL HISTORY: Dad is a demolition expert with the Navy Seals and mother is a housewife.

REVIEW OF SYSTEMS: Negative for 10 systems

PHYSICAL EXAMINATION:
Afebrile HR: 68/min RR: 24/min, BP: 145/98, Weight: 45 Kg (50%), Ht: 150 cm (50%)

HEENT:	Clear
Chest:	Clear
Heart:	Regular rate and rhythm with a 2/6 systolic ejection murmur along the second intercostal space to the right of the sternum. A bruit is audible along the posterior aspect of the chest.
Abdomen:	Soft without masses
Genitalia:	Normal male
Skin:	Without lesions
Extremities:	Clear
Neuro:	Nonfocal

You tell his mother you need to get an ECG and chest x-ray; she gets angry but finally agrees.

Chest x-ray:	Rib notching is noted on the left side of the chest
ECG:	Left axis deviation with left ventricular hypertrophy

Which of the following is the most likely cause of his hypertension?

     A. Essential hypertension
     B. Pheochromocytoma
     C. Caffeine-induced
     D. Ventricular septal defect
     E. Coarctation of the aorta

118.

A mother brings you her 6-month-old daughter with a history of cyanotic episodes. Upon taking the history, you learn that, when the baby gets upset, she will turn blue. Once she quits crying, her color returns to normal. You obtain the following history:

PRENATAL HISTORY:	No problems, prenatal care started at 4 months
NATAL HISTORY:	Normal spontaneous vaginal delivery with a birth weight of 3.5 Kg
HOSPITALIZATIONS:	None
IMMUNIZATIONS:	Up to date
ALLERGIES:	None
MEDICATIONS:	None
SURGERY:	None
DIET:	Breastfeeding only
FAMILY HISTORY:	Two other siblings alive and well; dad has hypertension and mom has fibromyalgia.
SOCIAL HISTORY:	The patient lives with her mother and father and sleeps in her own room.
REVIEW OF SYSTEMS:	Negative for 10 systems

PHYSICAL EXAMINATION:
Afebrile HR: 110/min, RR: 28/min, Weight: 6.4 Kg (50%), Ht: 64 cm (50%)

HEENT:	Clear
Chest:	Clear
Heart:	Regular rate and rhythm with a 3/6 systolic ejection murmur along the third intercostal space to the left of the sternum
Abdomen:	Soft without masses
Genitalia:	Normal female
Skin:	Without lesions
Extremities:	Clear
Neuro:	Nonfocal

You obtain a chest x-ray and ECG because of the murmur and cyanotic episodes.

Chest x-ray: Decreased pulmonary markings
ECG: Right ventricular hypertrophy

Which of the following is the most likely diagnosis?

    A. Severe pulmonary stenosis
    B. Tetralogy of Fallot
    C. Eisenmenger's complex
    D. Ventricular septal defect
    E. Tricuspid atresia

119.

You are called to evaluate a baby who is found to be extremely cyanotic soon after birth. You speak to the mother who tells you she had no real problems during pregnancy, except for a urinary tract infection at 6-months gestation. She was followed with prenatal care starting at 2-months gestation. This is her first baby, but she has felt that everything was fine. There is no family history of heart disease but there is for hypertension. She is worried and wants to know what you think.

PHYSICAL EXAMINATION:
Afebrile HR: 140/min, RR: 32/min, weight: 3.4 Kg, (50%), Ht: 53 cm (50%)

HEENT:	Cyanotic around the lips
Chest:	Clear
Heart:	Regular rate and rhythm with a 3/6 holosystolic murmur best heard at the left lower sternal border
Abdomen:	Soft with a 3-vessel cord
Genitalia:	Normal female
Skin:	Without lesions
Extremities:	Clear
Neuro:	Nonfocal

You obtain a chest x-ray and ECG.

Chest x-ray:	Elevated apex of the heart
ECG:	Right atrial and left ventricular hypertrophy

Which of the following is the most likely cardiac lesion?

- A. Tricuspid atresia
- B. Transposition of the great vessels
- C. Truncus arteriosus
- D. Tetralogy of Fallot
- E. Total anomalous pulmonary venous return

120.

A 2-year-old girl just moved to town and presents to you in the ER with a chief complaint of a draining right ear. You obtain the following history:

NATAL HISTORY:	Repeat c-section to a 32-year-old G3P3 for failure to progress. Birthweight was 3.5 kg
HOSPITALIZATIONS:	None
IMMUNIZATIONS:	Up to date
ALLERGIES:	None
MEDICATIONS:	None
SURGERY:	None
DIET:	Normal for age
DEVELOPMENT:	Sat at 9 months, walked at 20 months
FAMILY HISTORY:	Two other siblings alive and well; dad has a history of a ventricular septal defect, corrected at one year of age, and mom has problems with depression.
SOCIAL HISTORY:	Dad works as a short-order cook, and mom is an exotic dancer.
REVIEW OF SYSTEMS:	Mother states that this girl has not grown or developed as fast as her other two children.

PHYSICAL EXAMINATION:
Afebrile HR: 84/min, RR: 28/min, weight: 9.0 kg (< 5 %), Ht: 80 cm (< 5%)

HEENT:	Purulent drainage from the right ear canal
Chest:	Scattered crackles throughout the chest
Heart:	Regular rate and rhythm with a 2/6 systolic ejection murmur along the second intercostal space to the left of the sternum, with a widely split second heart sound and a mild diastolic rumble
Abdomen:	Soft with the liver palpable 3 centimeters below the right costal margin
Genitalia:	Normal female
Extremities:	No cyanosis, clubbing, or edema
Skin:	Without lesions
Extremities:	Clear
Neuro:	Nonfocal

You obtain a chest x-ray and ECG because of the murmur and rumble.

Chest x-ray:	Large right atrium and right ventricle with increased vascular markings and a wide mediastinum
ECG:	Right ventricular hypertrophy

Which of the following is the most likely diagnosis?

A. Atrial septal defect (ASD)
B. Total anomalous pulmonary venous return (TAPVR)
C. Tricuspid atresia
D. Ventricular septal defect (VSD)
E. Atrioventricular canal

121.

A 4-week-old male is brought to your office, whom your partner saw in the newborn period. He presents to you for his health supervision check since your partner is out of town. Mother states he is doing well. He eats 3–4 ounces every 3–4 hours of 20 cal/ounce formula. Mother is happy with everything, but this is her first child.

PRENATAL HISTORY:	A nurse midwife, starting at 16-weeks gestation, followed mother, who had problems with gestational diabetes. She is a 38-year-old G1P1.
NATAL HISTORY:	Normal spontaneous vaginal delivery with a birthweight of 3.4 Kg
HOSPITALIZATIONS:	None
IMMUNIZATIONS:	Hepatitis B #1 at birth
ALLERGIES:	None known
MEDICATIONS:	None
SURGERY:	Circumcision prior to leaving the hospital
FAMILY HISTORY:	There is hypertension and insulin-dependent diabetes mellitus on both sides of the family.
SOCIAL HISTORY:	Dad is 45 and the executive at a large bank; mother is an executive administrator at a local hospital.
REVIEW OF SYSTEMS:	Negative for 10 systems

PHYSICAL EXAMINATION:
Afebrile HR: 145/minute, RR: 26/min, weight: 4 Kg (75%), length: 55 cm (75%)

HEENT:	Flat face with slanted palpebral fissures and speckled irises
Chest:	Clear
Heart:	Regular rate and rhythm and without a murmur
Abdomen:	Soft with no hepatosplenomegaly
Genitalia:	Normal male with bilateral descended testes
Extremities:	Short, broad hands with hypoplasia of the middle phalanx of the 5th digit bilaterally
Skin:	Normal
Neuro:	Nonfocal examination but somewhat hypotonic tone

Which of the following cardiac defects should be investigated in this child?

A. Tetralogy of Fallot
B. Atrioventricular canal
C. Atrial septal defect
D. Ventricular septal defect
E. Coarctation of the aorta

122.

A 12-year-old male presents to your office for evaluation of a murmur. This family just moved to the area and presented to a local family medicine physician who heard the murmur and referred him to you for evaluation. Mother states he is an active young man but has always been rather small for his size. You obtain the following history:

NATAL HISTORY:	Born at 33 weeks to a 26-year-old G3P3 by vaginal delivery. The delivery was complicated by prolonged rupture of membranes and maternal chorioamnionitis. The baby was hospitalized for 2 weeks but only required oxygen by hood.
HOSPITALIZATIONS:	Pneumonia at 4 years
ALLERGIES:	Amoxicillin with a rash
IMMUNIZATIONS:	Up to date
SURGERY:	Inguinal hernia repair at 10 months, PE tubes at 18 months and a T&A at 36 months
DEVELOPMENT:	Normal
FAMILY HISTORY:	2 other siblings both alive and well. There is cancer on both sides of the family.
SOCIAL HISTORY:	He is in the 6th grade but usually keeps to himself. He is a B–C student.
REVIEW OF SYSTEMS:	Negative for 10 systems

PHYSICAL EXAMINATION:
Afebrile HR: 72/min, RR: 20/min, BP: 84/54, weight: 30 Kg (5%), height: 130 cm (< 5%)

HEENT:	Downward slanted palpebral fissures, bilateral ptosis and micrognathia, prominent webbing of the neck
Chest:	Pectus excavatum with clear breath sounds bilaterally
Heart:	Regular rate and rhythm with a 4/6 crescendo-decrescendo systolic murmur with a palpable thrill at the second left intercostal space
Abdomen:	Soft with no masses
Genitalia:	Only one testes is palpable
Skin:	Normal
Extremities:	Cubitus valgus
Neuro:	Nonfocal

Which of the following cardiac lesions is most likely?

    A. Coarctation of the aorta
    B. Aortic stenosis
    C. Mitral valve prolapse
    D. Tricuspid regurgitation
    E. Pulmonary valvular stenosis

123.

You are working at the after-hours clinic when a family arrives with a 4-year-old female for you to evaluate. The parents brought her in because she fell and cut her arm, and they wanted to know whether she might need stitches. You obtain the following history:

NATAL HISTORY:	Born at term without complications
HOSPITALIZATIONS:	None
ALLERGIES:	None
IMMUNIZATIONS:	Up to date
SURGERY:	None
DEVELOPMENT:	Normal
FAMILY HISTORY:	1 other sibling who is alive and well. There is hypertension and learning disabilities on mom's side of the family.
SOCIAL HISTORY:	She is in daycare since both mom and dad work at the local air force base.
REVIEW OF SYSTEMS:	Negative for 10 systems

PHYSICAL EXAMINATION:
Afebrile HR: 80/min, RR: 22/min, weight: 13 Kg (5%), height: 95 cm (< 5%)

HEENT:	Micrognathia, prominent webbing of the neck, and a high arched palate
Chest:	Broad chest with widely spaced nipples
Heart:	Regular rate and rhythm without murmurs, clicks, or rubs
Abdomen:	Soft with no masses
Genitalia:	Normal female
Skin:	2-centimeter superficial incision of the left forearm
Extremities:	Cubitus valgus and hyperconvex fingernails
Neuro:	Nonfocal

Which of the following cardiac abnormalities is most likely?

- A. Dilated aortic root
- B. Coarctation of the aorta
- C. Aortic stenosis
- D. Non-stenotic bicuspid aortic valve
- E. Mitral valve prolapse

124.

You are covering your partner's practice while he is on vacation. Your partner is very active in the community and works with patients who have special needs. The school calls you to come evaluate a new child who has been sent to them. This child has recently moved to the area after being placed in foster care. The past medical history is scant, but this is what you know about the 6-year-old child.

HOSPITALIZATIONS:	At 6 months for bronchiolitis
ALLERGIES:	None
IMMUNIZATIONS:	Withheld all DTaP vaccines due to developmental problems
SURGERIES:	None
DIET:	Normal for age
MEDICATIONS:	A "blue pill" for behavioral problems
FAMILY HISTORY:	None available
SOCIAL HISTORY:	Patient placed with child welfare due to neglect
REVIEW OF SYSTEMS:	Negative for 10 systems

PHYSICAL EXAMINATION:
Afebrile HR: 74/min, RR: 22/min, weight: 18 kg (10%), height: 110 cm (10%)

HEENT:	Round face with full cheeks, flattened bridge of the nose, long upper lip, and a stellate pattern in the iris bilaterally
Chest:	Clear
Heart:	Regular rate and rhythm with a 2/6 systolic ejection murmur along the sternal border
Abdomen:	Soft without masses
Genitalia:	Normal male with bilateral descended testes
Skin:	Without lesions
Extremities:	No cyanosis, clubbing, or edema
Neuro:	Patient is obviously mentally retarded but is very personable and happy. The rest of his exam is nonfocal.

You tell the school the child is doing well but has a murmur that needs to be better evaluated.

Which of the following cardiac lesions does this child most likely have?

   A. Supravalvular aortic stenosis
   B. Pulmonary stenosis
   C. Ventricular septal defect
   D. Atrial septal defect
   E. Atrioventricular canal

DERMATOLOGY

125.

A 14-year-old female is concerned because "clumps of hair come out" every time she combs her hair or washes it in the shower. On exam, she is noted to have diffuse thinning of the scalp hair, especially where she parts her hair down the middle. No associated scaling, erythema, or pustules are evident; and she reports that her scalp does not itch. She was hospitalized 3 months previously with a peritonsillar abscess that required drainage, followed by a 4-day hospital stay because of excessive bleeding following surgery. A diagnostic evaluation at that time revealed no evidence of a bleeding diathesis.

Here is a photograph of her thinning hair:

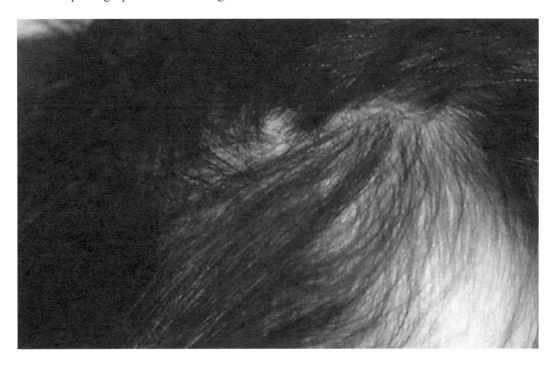

Which of the following is the most appropriate next step in the treatment of this patient?

   A. Obtain a scraping from her scalp for fungal and bacterial cultures.
   B. Begin treatment with oral griseofulvin.
   C. Reassure the patient that the condition is temporary, and that her hair will begin to thicken and return to normal over a several month period.
   D. Inform the patient that she is likely unaware that she is twisting and pulling her hair, and investigate further for a cause underlying anxiety/stress.
   E. Begin treatment with corticosteroid injections along the part line.

126.

A 17-year-old female being treated for a urinary tract infection presents complaining of a rapidly worsening rash first noted 24 hours earlier. On exam, multiple erythematous macules associated with vesicular and bullous lesions, some of which show evidence of associated necrosis and denuded skin, are noted. Intense erythema of both conjunctiva associated with photophobia is noted, as is hemorrhagic crusting along the lips and in the nares.

Which of the following is most likely responsible for the patient's findings?

    A. Trimethoprim-sulfamethoxazole
    B. Amoxicillin/clavulanic acid
    C. Nitrofurantoin
    D. Cefdinir
    E. Cefixime

127.

A 12-year-old boy presents with a history of a worsening rash over the last 10 days. On physical examination, multiple, discrete 2–8 mm in diameter, "drop-like" papules with a pinkish hue are noted, some of which have an associated fine, scaly appearance. Lesions are most prominent on the trunk and proximal extremities. The palms and soles are spared.

Which of the following conditions is most likely to be associated with this disorder?

    A. Sensorineural hearing loss and chronic renal insufficiency
    B. Recurrent episodes of skin and soft tissue abscesses
    C. Sore throat within the preceding 2–3 weeks
    D. Recurrent episodes of hematuria following upper respiratory infection
    E. Autoimmune thyroiditis

128.

The foster parents of a 5-year-old girl express their concern about her hair loss. She has been in foster care for the last 2 weeks after being removed from her natural parents due to medical neglect and physical abuse. She is described as "an anxious child" but appears to be comfortable with her foster parents. They are unaware of associated underlying medical problems and deny that she takes daily medications or has any allergies. On physical exam, she has multiple linear areas with irregular borders of partial hair loss. The remaining hairs are broken off at various lengths and appear firmly rooted in the scalp. There is no associated erythema, scaling, or folliculitis.

Here is a photograph of her scalp:

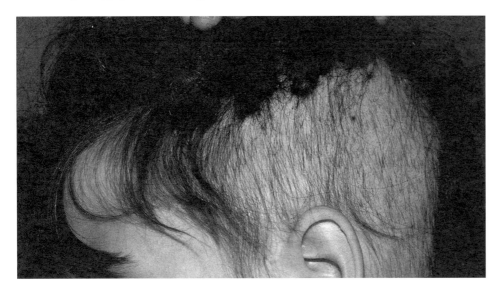

Which of the following is the most appropriate next step in the treatment of this child?

A. Oral griseofulvin 25 mg/kg/day for 8 weeks.
B. Topical ketoconazole 2% cream twice daily for 2 weeks.
C. Oral cephalexin 250 mg twice daily for 2 weeks.
D. Inform the parents that no medications are indicated.
E. Topical 0.1% triamcinolone cream in combination with topical ketoconazole 2% cream twice daily for 2 weeks.

129.

A 5-year-old African-American boy presents with a 2-day history of a pruritic rash that began on his face, neck, and scalp before spreading to his trunk. He is otherwise well with no history of associated systemic complaints. Three weeks earlier, he was started on griseofulvin for treatment of tinea capitis. On physical examination, small lichenoid flesh-colored papules are noted on the scalp, neck, face, and trunk.

Which of the following represents the most likely etiology of the rash?

A. Pityriasis rosea
B. Scabies
C. Allergic drug reaction
D. Autoeczematization ("id" reaction)
E. Viral exanthem

130.

A 16-year-old male is concerned that his "ringworm infection" is not improving. He has applied topical antifungal creams twice daily during the preceding two weeks but states that the lesions continue to enlarge. He is otherwise well. He does take ibuprofen daily for knee pain associated with Osgood-Schlatter disease. He has been advised to stop playing basketball but refuses to do so. On physical examination, there are several 2.5–3.5 cm annular lesions on the dorsal surface of his left leg (see figure below). The lesions have prominent raised borders, which surround a smooth, firm, and slightly depressed center.

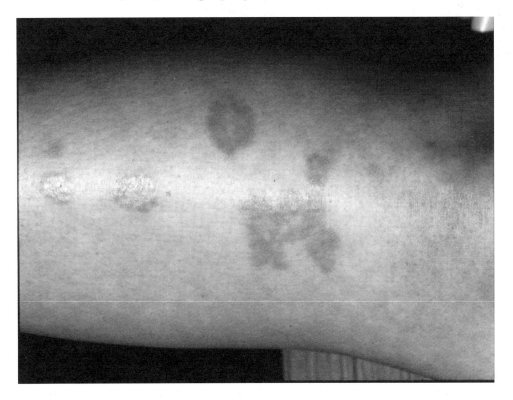

Which of the following is the most appropriate next step in the treatment of this patient?

    A. A punch biopsy of the lesion(s).
    B. Laboratory testing for ANA and antibodies to double-stranded DNA.
    C. Advise the patient to use acetaminophen rather than ibuprofen for pain due to a possible drug reaction as a cause of the lesions.
    D. Discontinue topical treatment and reassure the patient that the lesions will slowly resolve without further intervention.
    E. Laboratory testing for RPR.

131.

The mother of a 4-year-old African-American male presents with the concern that her son has recently developed "sores on his scalp." On physical examination, there are several erythematous, scaling patches where hair has broken away flush with the scalp causing a "black dot" appearance. One patch is associated with a large, very tender boggy nodule (see figure below). Several tender, posterior cervical lymph nodes are also present. Palpation of both the nodule and lymph nodes produces significant discomfort.

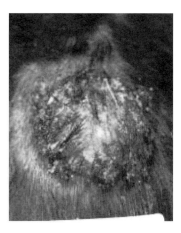

Which of the following represents the most appropriate treatment in patients with this disorder?

    A. Selenium sulfide
    B. Both oral griseofulvin and cephalexin
    C. Oral cephalexin
    D. Topical nystatin
    E. Both oral griseofulvin and prednisone

132.

A 15-year-old male presents for follow-up five months after beginning oral antibiotics in addition to topical treatment for acne. On physical examination, his lesions appear to have worsened. A decision is made to begin the patient on isotretinoin.

Which of the following laboratory tests should be obtained prior to onset of treatment and at regular intervals?

    A. Amylase and lipase
    B. BUN and creatinine
    C. Liver function tests
    D. Thyroid function tests
    E. Insulin levels

133.

During a physical examination in the newborn nursery, a 7-pound, 2-ounce male born by an uncomplicated vaginal delivery at 38-weeks gestation is noted to have a slightly raised, solitary, yellowish-tan, hairless plaque on the scalp just above the right ear. On palpation, it is firm with an "oily" and "velvety" consistency.

Here is a picture:

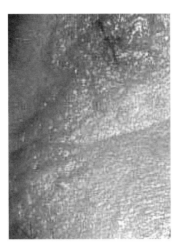

Which of the following is the most appropriate treatment of this lesion?

    A. Elective excision prior to puberty
    B. Twice-daily application of a hydrocortisone cream
    C. Topical destruction of the lesion with trichloroacetic acid
    D. Tzanck smear to examine for multinucleated giant cells
    E. Wright stain to examine for eosinophilia

134.

A 9-year-old boy with a history of atopic dermatitis presents with a 2-day history of "painful swelling" at the tips of several fingers. On physical examination, a fluid-filled, tense blister with surrounding erythema is located over the volar fat pad on the distal portion of both the third and fourth fingers of the right hand.

Which of the following is the most common cause of these clinical findings?

    A. Group A beta-hemolytic streptococcus
    B. Herpes simplex virus
    C. *Staphylococcus aureus*
    D. *Pseudomonas aeruginosa*
    E. *Pasteurella multocida*

135.

A 15-month-old girl, who was recently adopted from an orphanage in Thailand, presents with a history of a mildly pruritic rash. She was first evaluated 10 days ago after her adoptive parents first noticed the rash. She was diagnosed with a "viral rash" and treated symptomatically. She has otherwise been well with the exception of an intermittent low-grade fever. On physical examination, multiple small pinkish-brown papular and papulovesicular lesions are symmetrically distributed on the extensor portions of both the forearms (see figure below) and legs. Similar lesions are also present on the buttocks, face, and, to a lesser extent, the trunk. None of the lesions are scaly.

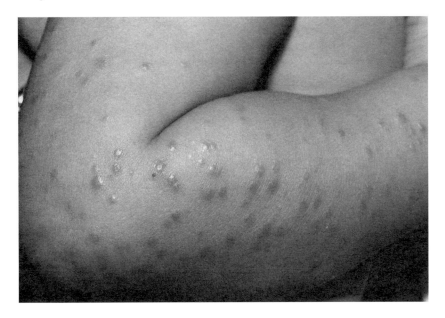

Which of the following is a known cause of this type of rash?

    A. Adenovirus
    B. Hepatitis C virus
    C. *Treponema pallidum*
    D. Hepatitis B virus
    E. Group A coxsackievirus

136.

A 19-year-old male with a history of "psoriasis" presents to the infirmary at his college. He is visibly distraught. After being consoled, he states that he "knows he has some terrible venereal disease" because of several lesions on his penis that he discovered while showering. He has been sexually active with several female partners over the previous 6 months and has used a condom only intermittently. On physical examination, he has 8–10 violaceous papules on the glans penis. Upon further examination, discrete, shiny, polygonal scaling erythematous papules are noted on the wrist and flexor surfaces of the forearm which, by history, are intensely pruritic and sometimes painful.

Which of the following is most likely to be identified upon further examination?

A. Displacement of the lens on slit lamp examination
B. Positive direct fluorescent antibody test for herpes simplex virus on fluid taken from lesions on the glans penis
C. Patches of smooth, circular complete hair loss
D. Decreased levels of serum ceruloplasmin
E. Whitish lace-like lesions on the lateral buccal mucosa

137.

A 4-year-old girl who was diagnosed with "chickenpox" 15 days ago presents with her parents, who are concerned that their daughter continues to develop new lesions. They describe that she "seems to keep getting new groups of itchy bumps." On physical examination, her most recent lesions appear as 2–4 mm rounded, reddish-brown macules and papules. Older lesions, some of which are beginning to crust, are both vesicular and necrotic in appearance. Lesions are most prominent on the trunk and are symmetrically distributed over the proximal thighs and flexor surfaces of the arms.

Here is a picture of her upper leg:

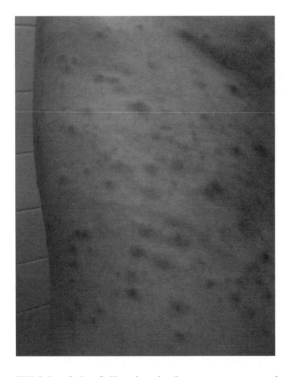

Which of the following is the most appropriate treatment?

A. Topical corticosteroids
B. Systemic corticosteroids
C. Oral erythromycin
D. Oral cephalexin
E. Intravenous immunoglobulin

138.

Following an uncomplicated term vaginal delivery, a Caucasian girl weighing 7 pounds, 1 ounce is noted to have large areas of erythematous skin erosion. In addition, there are several large intact blisters on the hands and feet and a large denuded area over the left buttocks and lower posterior trunk. The base of the umbilical cord is also intensely erythematous.

Which of the following diagnostic procedures is most likely to reveal the etiology of this patient's skin lesions?

   A. Skin biopsy
   B. Blood culture
   C. Tzanck smear
   D. Culture of fluid aspirated from an intact blister
   E. Rapid plasma regain (RPR)

139.

A 4-year-old girl is brought to the ER by her babysitter after she noticed a rash on her right hand and right leg. On physical examination, blisters and irregular linear areas of purplish erythema are present on the right hand. Linear streaks of purplish erythema and hyperpigmentation with bizarre patterning are noted on the right leg with additional associated blistering. There is no history of known trauma or allergies. The patient takes no daily medications. The patient, her parents, and the babysitter returned from Mexico the day prior to presentation, having spent the last several days at a beach resort. The babysitter reports that, while at the beach, she was careful to liberally apply sunscreen and that the patient had only "waded in the water up to her knees," always accompanied by an adult.

Which of the following is the most likely cause of this patient's lesions?

   A. Non-accidental trauma
   B. Jellyfish sting
   C. Sunburn
   D. Phytophotodermatitis
   E. Stinging nematocyst of a cnidarian larva

140.

You are called to evaluate a newborn. On exam, you notice the port wine stain over the entire right side of the face. The remainder of the exam is normal.

Which of the following evaluations is necessary?

   A. Imaging of the brain and ophthalmologic evaluation
   B. ANA testing
   C. Chromosomal analysis
   D. Reassurance to the parents that their child will develop normally
   E. Immediate laser surgery to the face

141.

You see a 17-year-old male for a rash. He has had no fever and does not appear ill. His mother reports that he had ringworm on his back about a week ago, but that seems better. He woke up this morning and now has the rash on his arms, back, and stomach. On physical examination, he is alert and looks well. His temperature is 99° F. He has slight nasal congestion and multiple small, oval, scaling pink papules on his trunk. You notice that these papules follow the lines of skin cleavage. Otherwise, his exam is unremarkable.

Here is a picture of the rash:

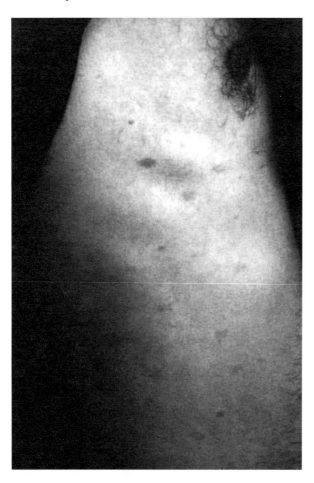

Which of the following is the most appropriate next step in treatment?

    A. You refer him immediately to a dermatologist.
    B. You recommend that he apply a topic antifungal cream 3 times per day.
    C. You tell him he should absolutely avoid the sun.
    D. You start him on a 10-day course of amoxicillin.
    E. You reassure him that this is a self-limited process and that sunlight may help to accelerate remission.

142.

You are seeing a well newborn infant for a routine checkup at 3 days of age. Pregnancy and delivery were both normal with no complications. She is nursing well and acting normal. Mother is concerned about heat rash because the infant broke out in a rash the day before.

On physical examination, the infant is alert and well hydrated. Everything appears normal, but she does have a rash of multiple yellow papules and pustules surrounded by large, erythematous rings mainly on the trunk (see figure below); but a few are on the face.

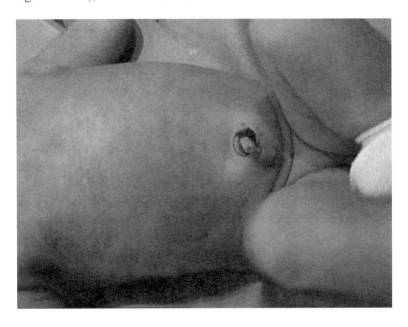

Which of the following is the most likely diagnosis?

    A. Transient neonatal pustular melanosis
    B. Seborrheic dermatitis
    C. Erythema toxicum neonatorum (ETN)
    D. Acrodermatitis enteropathica
    E. Miliaria crystallina

143.

A 16-year-old female presents with a 3-year history of predominantly open and closed comedones of the face, chest, and back. Close inspection reveals an occasional pustule and postinflammatory macules.

Which of the following is the most helpful medication for her type of acne vulgaris?

    A. Topical tretinoin
    B. Topical antibiotic
    C. Topical sulfacetamide lotion
    D. Systemic tetracycline
    E. Topical interferon-alpha

144.

A 17-year-old African-American female gives a 4-month history of tender nodules on pre-tibial surfaces associated with arthralgias (see figure below of similar lesions in a Caucasian girl). The remainder of the examination is normal. Biopsy of one of the nodules shows a septal panniculitis. Her chest x-ray shows bilateral hilar adenopathy. Trans-bronchial lung biopsy reveals non-caseating granuloma.

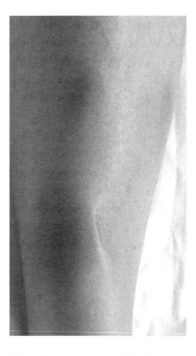

You diagnose sarcoidosis.

Which of the following do the lesions on her legs represent?

    A. Unrecalled trauma
    B. Cutaneous sarcoidosis
    C. A viral exanthem
    D. Erythema nodosum
    E. Erythema marginatum

145.

A 5-year-old girl was well until 2 weeks ago when she sustained mosquito bites to her face, which she has been scratching. Today the lesions are erythematous and covered with honey-colored crusts (see figure below).

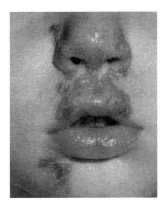

Which of the following is the most likely diagnosis?

A. Impetigo vulgaris
B. Erythema nodosum
C. Acne vulgaris
D. A drug eruption
E. Vitiligo

146.

A 20-year-old college student comes to see you because of vesicles on sun-exposed areas, which have been present episodically for 7 years. He has used alcohol to excess for many years. He takes no medications and has not seen a physician for many years. Your evaluation confirms a diagnosis of porphyria cutanea tarda (PCT).

Which of the following other diagnoses should you also consider?

A. Paraneoplastic pemphigus
B. Urinary tract infection
C. Acanthosis nigricans
D. Hepatitis C
E. Hepatitis D

147.

A 13-year-old male comes to you because of a diffuse scaling eruption that almost completely covers his entire body. He reports that the symptoms began shortly after he began to take phenytoin for a seizure disorder. Your examination shows confluent erythematous patches with contiguous scale, generalized lymphadenopathy, and hepatomegaly. Laboratory testing reveals peripheral eosinophilia.

Exfoliative dermatitis may be associated with all of the following <u>except</u>:

A. Drugs
B. Atopic dermatitis
C. Herpetic infections
D. Lymphoma
E. Solid tumors

148.

An 11-year-old girl is seen for evaluation of rash. She was in her usual excellent state of health until 1 week ago while on vacation in Hawaii. At that time, she developed frequency and dysuria. Her mother treated her with "left-over antibiotics." Physical examination shows severe sunburn.

Which of the following is the most likely antibiotic that she was given?
A. Amoxicillin/clavulanate
B. Nitrofurantoin
C. Norfloxacin
D. Erythromycin
E. Tetracycline

149.

A 17-year-old works in a restaurant as a dishwasher. She has to wash her hands multiple times in a day—likely exceeding 30–40 episodes daily. She has noted a small skin lesion between the 3rd interdigital web of her left hand (see figure below). It is erosive in character.

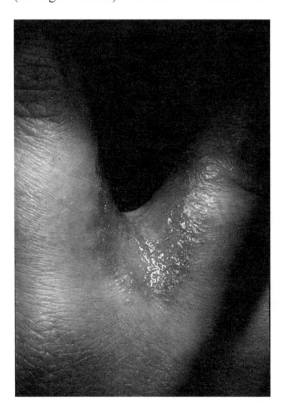

Which of the following is the most likely etiology?

   A. Cutaneous candidal infection
   B. Cutaneous bacterial infection
   C. Human papillomavirus infection
   D. Psoriasis
   E. Acanthosis nigricans

150.

A 15-year-old dishwasher presents with scaling of her hands. Recently, she has also noted vesicle formation. She has always had dry scaly lesions on her hands, and they remit and worsen over time. Sometimes the lesions are quite painful. She never had asthma or skin problems as a child. Recently, she noted that the small vesicles on the sides of her fingers itch quite a bit.

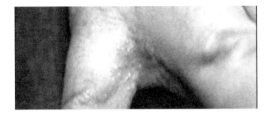

Which of the following is the most likely diagnosis?

   A. Dyshidrotic eczema
   B. Herpes simplex I
   C. Atopic dermatitis
   D. Lichen planus
   E. Varicella zoster

151.

A 13-year-old girl presents with a history of having multiple telangiectasias on her lips, face, feet, and in her nail beds. The telangiectasias are "spider-like"—when you pull the overlying skin over an individual lesion, a central area with radiating vessels is noted. Many members of her family have similar findings, she says.

Here are her lips showing the "spider-like" telangiectasia:

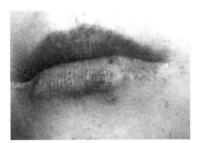

Which of the following is the most likely diagnosis?

A. CREST
B. Actinically damaged skin
C. Osler-Rendu-Weber disease
D. SLE
E. Scleroderma

152.

A 17-year-old male homosexual presents with a diffuse maculopapular rash over his trunk, head, neck, palms, and even his soles! He has had generalized lymphadenopathy for a few days. He has a history of a painless lesion on his anus about 2 months ago.

Which of the following is the most likely diagnosis?

A. SLE
B. Bacterial endocarditis
C. Syphilis
D. HIV
E. Herpes simplex

153.

An 18-year-old pop singer visits you for his yearly checkup. Physical examination is unremarkable except for white patches involving his face, hands, trunk, anus, and genitalia. The white spots have been present for several years.

Here is a photograph of his hand:

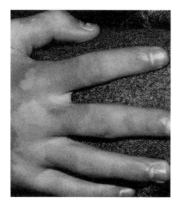

This condition has been associated with all of the following except:

A. Folate deficiency
B. Diabetes mellitus
C. Vitamin B_{12} deficiency
D. Hyperthyroidism
E. Hypothyroidism

EMERGENCY MEDICINE

154.

An institutionalized mentally challenged 6-year-old boy with a 36-hour history of gastroenteritis suddenly becomes very agitated and appears frightened. He points to his mouth and appears unable to fully open it. His speech is slurred, and he is drooling excessively. His head and neck are positioned to the left, and it appears difficult for him to follow to the right.

Which of the following is the most likely cause of his symptoms?

A. Ingestion of a foreign body
B. Partial complex seizure
C. Epiglottitis
D. Adverse reaction to promethazine hydrochloride (Phenergan®)
E. Uremia associated with hemolytic uremic syndrome

155.

Following a tonsillectomy and adenoidectomy, a 6-year-old boy is found to have a temperature of 105.8°F and reddish-brown urine. Surgery was uneventful, although he was initially difficult to intubate because of rigid clenching of the masseter muscles during induction. He soon develops an irregular heart rhythm and hypotension and is placed back on a ventilator.

Which of the following is the most likely cause of his symptoms?

A. Aspiration pneumonia
B. Renal vein thrombosis
C. Coagulopathy
D. An inhalation anesthetic
E. Gram-negative septicemia

156.

A 5-month-old boy, recently adopted from Russia, presents for evaluation. His adoptive parents know little about his natural mother, except that she did take an unknown medication throughout her pregnancy. On physical examination, his head circumference is in the 3rd percentile, height is at the 15th percentile, and weight is at the 65th percentile. He has evidence of midfacial hypoplasia associated with a short nose, with a broad, depressed bridge and epicanthal folds. He has an unrepaired cleft lip and palate. Coarse hair and hirsutism, finger-like thumbs, and hypoplasia of the distal phalanges and nail beds are also noted.

Which of the following medications is the most likely cause of this patient's dysmorphic findings?

A. Propranolol
B. Phenytoin
C. Valproate
D. Hydralazine
E. Captopril

157.

A 16-year-old boy is transported to the emergency room after he was found in a confused state while lying on the bathroom floor at his high school. He appears disoriented and complains of headache, shortness of breath, and dizziness. He is noted to have a bluish-gray discoloration of the skin and mucus membranes. Arterial blood, which appears reddish-brown in color, is obtained, and it reveals a normal arterial oxygen tension (PaO_2).

Which of the following substances is the most likely cause of this patient's symptoms?

    A. Marijuana
    B. Lysergic acid diethylamide
    C. Phencyclidine
    D. Methylenedioxymethamphetamine
    E. Amyl nitrite

158.

A 15-year-old boy presents for evaluation due to a decrease in school performance over the previous 6 months. Once a "straight-A" student, he is now failing three classes and, according to his parents, "just doesn't seem to care anymore." He has also quit the high school soccer team and has established a new group of friends who are known to be involved with drugs.

Which of the following findings on physical examination is associated with chronic use of marijuana?

    A. Gynecomastia
    B. Bradycardia
    C. Hepatosplenomegaly
    D. Hypertrichosis on the face and trunk
    E. Purplish striae on the abdomen and thighs

159.

A 17-year-old female is transported to the emergency room after being found sitting alone in a bathroom "drooling and talking like she was crazy." She and several of her friends "snuck into a party" and were just "hanging out drinking some wine coolers" when the patient's friends noticed she was missing. On exam, she is disoriented to time, place, and person; unable to recognize friends and family members; appears extremely anxious and frightened; and is drooling excessively. Her blood pressure is 70/38 and her pulse is 140 beats/minute. Her initial temperature is 102.2° F, but drops to 99.4° F within minutes. On cranial nerve testing, prominent nystagmus is noted. She is noted to have very brisk deep tendon reflexes with 2–3-beat clonus evident in the lower extremities.

Which of the following substances is the most likely cause of her clinical findings?

    A. Heroin
    B. Phencyclidine
    C. Cocaine
    D. Narcotic analgesics
    E. Toluene

160.

A 3-year-old boy presents to the emergency room after his mother noted him to be confused and disoriented when she checked on him while he and a friend were playing outside. On physical examination, he appears confused and is coughing, tearing, and drooling profusely. His temperature is 99.7° F, blood pressure 65/40, and heart rate 50. He vomits twice and is noted to be incontinent of urine.

Which of the following is the most likely cause of this patient's signs and symptoms?

- A. Epiglottitis
- B. Foreign-body aspiration
- C. Insecticide ingestion
- D. Postictal state
- E. Laryngotracheobronchitis

161.

A 2-year-old girl presents to the emergency room after she was found lying on the garage floor "choking and vomiting." On physical examination, she is lethargic and difficult to arouse. Unintentional poisoning is suspected.

Which of the following laboratory findings is most consistent with ingestion of car radiator antifreeze?

- A. Calcium oxalate crystals in the urine
- B. Red blood cell casts in the urine
- C. Elevated levels of serum amylase and lipase
- D. Hyperkalemia
- E. Hypomagnesemia

162.

The parents of a 3-year-old boy state that they were awakened by "noises and grunts" coming from their son's room. They go on to describe tonic-clonic seizure activity, which prompted immediate transport to the emergency room by EMS. On physical examination, there is no current seizure activity. He appears flushed and is extremely lethargic. Blood pressure is 70/30, heart rate 125, temperature 102.9° F. The pupils are dilated. An ECG shows a prolonged QT interval, widening of the QRS complex, and right bundle branch block.

Which one of the following substances did he most likely ingest?

- A. Propranolol
- B. Fluoxetine
- C. Digitalis
- D. Acetaminophen
- E. Amitriptyline

163.

A 10-year-old boy is bitten by a venomous snake while on an overnight camping trip with his Boy Scout troop.

Which of the following is the most appropriate management for him as arrangements are made for transport to a medical facility?

    A. Apply a constrictive tourniquet just above the site of the bite.
    B. Incise the area with two perpendicular incisions intersecting at the midline of the bite.
    C. Perform oral suction at the site of the bite for up to 5 minutes.
    D. Apply ice to the area of the bite.
    E. Cleanse the wound and immobilize the injured body part in a functional position below the level of the heart.

164.

A 15-year-old boy presents to the emergency room complaining of left eye swelling and pain associated with blurry vision. The evening prior to admission, he was involved in a "gang initiation," during which time he was assaulted by several rival gang members. He reports being hit in the face with a lead pipe. On physical examination, there is evidence of left-sided periorbital edema with prominent ecchymosis.

Which of the following additional findings is most suggestive of an orbital floor blowout fracture?

    A. Hyphema
    B. Dilation of the pupil with only a sluggish reaction to light
    C. Restriction of upward gaze during testing of extraocular movements
    D. Leakage of clear fluid from the nose
    E. Left hemotympanum associated with a perforation

165.

A 4-year-old girl presents to the emergency room with a 36-hour history of vomiting and diarrhea. Her parents report that she has continued to worsen despite treatment with oral rehydrating fluids and an antiemetic obtained from their pediatrician. On physical examination, she appears dehydrated and requires treatment with intravenous fluids. Two hours after arrival at the emergency room, she suddenly becomes anxious and very agitated, screaming that she cannot swallow and complaining of severe neck and back pain. On physical examination, she is noted to have torticollis, muscle rigidity, deviation of the eyes to the left, and trismus.

Which of the following is the most appropriate next step in the treatment of this patient?

    A. Administer diphenhydramine.
    B. Obtain serum calcium, magnesium, and phosphorus levels.
    C. Administer phenobarbital.
    D. Obtain a urine drug screen.
    E. Obtain a CT scan of the head.

166.

A 30-month-old boy is transported to the emergency room after his mother found him "eating pills from a bottle of baby aspirin." He routinely takes daily low-dose aspirin due to a history of a coronary artery aneurysm identified during a recent hospitalization for Kawasaki disease.

Which of the following laboratory manifestations is most likely to be identified in this patient?

A. Metabolic alkalosis
B. Hypoglycemia during the early stage of salicylate intoxication, followed by hyperglycemia as poisoning progresses
C. A paradoxically acidic urine as poisoning progresses
D. A low anion-gap metabolic acidosis
E. Hyperkalemia

167.

A 17-year-old is transported to the emergency room after being found unconscious in his car after running off the road. Upon examination, he is lethargic but arousable. Vital signs are stable. He has multiple facial bruises, blood behind the left tympanic membrane, and continuous clear nasal discharge.

Which of the following findings is most likely to be present upon additional examination of this patient?

A. Absent breath sounds on the left
B. A displaced point of maximal impulse (PMI)
C. Asymmetric size of the pupils
D. Conjunctival hemorrhage
E. Postauricular ecchymosis

168.

A 16-year-old male is transported to the emergency room by several friends because he was "stumbling around like he was drunk" and complaining of "coughing, chest tightness, and difficulty breathing." The patient, however, denies recent intake of alcohol. He also complains of nausea, headache, dizziness, and lightheadedness. Vital signs include blood pressure of 136/80 mmHg, an irregularly irregular heart rate of 98 beats/minute, respiratory rate of 26 breaths/minute, and temperature of 99.8° F. The scleras are moderately injected. There are mild expiratory wheezes throughout both lung fields but no rales. Frequent ectopic beats are noted during cardiac examination. Soon after presentation, he becomes more difficult to arouse and experiences a generalized tonic-clonic seizure. Initial laboratory findings include a metabolic acidosis, hypokalemia, hematuria, and proteinuria.

Which of the following is the most likely cause of his symptoms?

A. Phencyclidine
B. Marijuana
C. Mescaline
D. d-lysergic acid diethylamide
E. Toluene

169.

The 21-year-old mother of a 5-year-old girl calls you in the middle of the night when you are on call. She was cleaning up after a party. One of her friends knocked the open container of drain cleaner off the cabinet. The drain cleaner splashed in the child's eye. The child is in significant pain.

Which of the following should you recommend?

A. Go directly to the emergency room.
B. Bring the child to see you in the office the following morning.
C. Call in a prescription for an antibiotic ophthalmic solution for the child to start using.
D. Lavage the eyes for about 15 minutes, then go directly to the emergency room.
E. Join the party at the mom's house and evaluate the child there.

170.

You go to the ER to meet a 5-year-old child who had drain cleaner accidentally splashed in her eye. The mother asks if you can also see the patient's 2-year-old half-sister. Apparently, while the mother was following your instructions to flush the eye of her 5-year-old with water, the 2-year-old was left unattended. She found the half-empty bottle of drain cleaner, which was left on the floor, and drank the remainder of the contents. The mother thinks she is okay but just wants her checked out since they are already there anyway. On exam, the 2-year-old has erythematous macules appearing on her face, concentrated around the mouth. The oral mucous membranes appear to have multiple abrasions with some swelling of the tongue.

Which of the following is the most appropriate next step?

A. Make the child NPO and refer for inpatient EGD.
B. Give the child some orange juice to drink to offset the alkali in the drain cleaner.
C. Give syrup of ipecac to induce vomiting.
D. Nasogastric tube lavage of the child's stomach.
E. Discharge the child and have her follow up in your office the next day.

171.

A 17-year-old boy "walks in" the ER for evaluation of an eye injury. He is the star of the high school baseball team and just came from a game, where he was hit in the eye by a pitch. He, of course, completed the game but now wants to get checked out. On exam, you notice bruising of the lower eyelid with limitation of upward gaze. There is some crepitus around the affected orbit. He has decreased sensation over the ipsilateral cheek and upper lip. The ipsilateral nares contain a small amount of blood. He wants to know if he can return to the field for the next game.

Which of the following is the most appropriate next step?

A. Refer to a neurologist.
B. Get x-rays and/or a CT scan of the orbit.
C. Check his CBC and ESR.
D. Apply ice to the affected area and give NSAIDs. Since the team is in the playoffs, he may return immediately to play.
E. Refer for ophthalmologic evaluation in the next week or so.

172.

You are seeing a 15-year-old previously healthy female who was found collapsed in her bedroom. She has had no recent illnesses or fever. She has been upset the last few days after her boyfriend broke up with her.

On physical examination, she is unresponsive with minimal respirations. BP 82/54. HR 52. Pupils are pinpoint, and she has decreased bowel sounds. Perfusion is adequate.

You provide respiratory support and place her on continuous ECG monitoring, which shows no arrhythmia at this time. Vascular access is established, and appropriate labs are sent, which confirm the diagnosis.

Which of the following treatments should you initiate?

    A. Supportive care only
    B. Activated charcoal
    C. Gastric lavage
    D. Syrup of ipecac
    E. Naloxone

173.

A 10-year-old from east Texas presents with a painful rash that started 4 hours ago. She noticed that her upper arm was hurting and lifted her sleeve to find a blue circular area. Shortly thereafter, she began feeling feverish with nausea and chills. She has been healthy and had no symptoms prior to a few hours ago.

On physical examination, temperature is 100° F. She appears to be a little uncomfortable but is stable. She has a 1.5 cm blue macule with surrounding inflammation.

Which of the following is the most appropriate management?

    A. Supportive care
    B. Amoxicillin-clavulanate
    C. Steroid injection
    D. Hydrocortisone
    E. Sunlight to the area

174.

You are evaluating a 12-year-old female who ingested at least twenty-five 500 mg tablets of acetaminophen 1 hour ago. She weighs approximately 50 kg; therefore, her dose was at least 250 mg/kg. Her mother thinks there could have been even more than 25 tablets in the bottle. No other medicines were in the house.

Presently, on physical examination, she is alert and in no discomfort or distress. Vital signs are stable, and she appears fine.

All of the following are true <u>except</u>:

A. AST is the earliest and most sensitive laboratory test of hepatotoxicity and is usually elevated by 24–36 hours.
B. A single dose of 150 mg/kg requires intervention.
C. You should get the first plasma level of acetaminophen at 2 hours post-ingestion to determine need for treatment.
D. N-acetyl-p-benzoquinone imine (NAPQI) is the metabolite that causes hepatic damage.
E. N-acetylcysteine (NAC) is most effective if administered within 8 hours of ingestion.

175.

You evaluate a 2-year-old female presenting with vomiting, diarrhea, and muscle twitches. She is very irritable. She has had no recent illnesses and no fever. You ask about possible exposures to drugs or toxins. The mother is unsure, because the child spent most of the day with her grandfather on his farm.

On physical examination, she is irritable, has miosis, tearing, salivation, sweating, muscular twitching, and loss of reflexes.

Which of the following is most likely?

A. Acetaminophen ingestion
B. Hydrocarbon ingestion
C. Ibuprofen ingestion
D. Organophosphate poisoning
E. Phenothiazine poisoning

176.

A 15-year-old motorcycle enthusiast is brought to the emergency room following a collision with a sport utility vehicle. He was trapped under the rear of the vehicle and was extracted after the Jaws of Life was brought in. He suffered severe injuries to his pelvis and legs and was rushed to the emergency room as soon as he was freed. In the ER, his initial blood pressure was 85/palpable with a heart rate of 136/minute. His blood pressure improved with 3 liters of normal saline and 4 units of blood. Further evaluation revealed multiple fractures of his pelvis and both tibias. His initial hemoglobin was 8.9 and hematocrit 28.4%, but his electrolytes, urinalysis, and liver function tests were normal. His BUN was 13 and serum creatinine was 1.0. Following an open reduction and fixation of both tibias, he was brought to the SICU for observation. The next day, the patient's urine output began to fall, and his serum creatinine rose to 2.9. His urinalysis revealed specific gravity of 1.010, pH of 5.5, 4+ blood, trace protein, 1–2 RBCs per high-power field, and 4–6 granular casts. A CPK was 25,500 with pending urine myoglobin. His heart rate began to slow, and an ECG demonstrated a rate of 45, with no P waves, and a widening of the QRS.

Which of the following is the best immediate step in the management of this patient?

A. Temporary pacemaker placement.
B. Administer sodium polystyrene sulfonate (Kayexalate®, Kionex®, SPS®) enemas.
C. Initiate dialysis therapy.
D. Administer calcium gluconate.
E. Perform fasciotomies.

177.

Which of the following is most frequently seen with kerosene ingestion?

A. Chemical pneumonitis
B. Aplastic anemia
C. Hepatitis
D. Coma
E. Seizures

178.

A 16-year-old female is admitted to the ICU after an emergency exploratory laparotomy for a ruptured ectopic pregnancy. She received 16 units of packed red cells in the OR, and a Swan-Ganz catheter was placed by anesthesia because they heard rales and were concerned about volume overload. On admission, she is in shock with a blood pressure of 70/30 mmHg and a hemoglobin of 5.0 g/dL. She is on mechanical ventilation in CMV mode with FiO_2 60%, PEEP 10 cm, Rate 20, and Tidal Volume 700 cc. Two additional units of packed cells were given on arrival to the ICU, and the blood pressure came up to 100/60 mmHg and the heart rate is 120 beats/minute. Post-transfusion labs reveal a hemoglobin of 7.0 g/dL, and the Swan-Ganz readings show a cardiac output of 10 L/min, pulmonary arterial "wedge" pressure of 12 mmHg, and a systemic vascular resistance of 600 dyne-sec-cm (low). The arterial blood gas now is PO_2 85 mmHg, PCO_2 44 mmHg, and pH 7.26.

Which of the following therapies is the most appropriate for continuing the resuscitation of this patient?

A. Increase the rate of the ventilator to increase the minute ventilation and lower the PCO_2.
B. Increase FiO_2 to 70%.
C. Transfuse 2 units of packed red blood cells.
D. Start dobutamine at 10 μg/kg/min to increase the cardiac output.
E. Start dopamine at 10 μg/kg/min to increase the systemic vascular resistance.

179.

A 17-year-old girl, with a history of end-stage renal disease on hemodialysis, presents to the emergency room with fever of 103° F, shaking chills, hypotension (70/50 mmHg), tachypnea, and tachycardia. Her dialysis graft site is erythematous and warm to the touch, and there is purulent drainage at a prior access site. A diagnosis of septic shock is made. The patient is given intravenous antibiotics and IV fluids, and arrangements are made to transfer her to the ICU with a vascular surgery consult to remove the hemodialysis graft. The intensivist meets the patient in the ER and immediately places a Swan-Ganz catheter because of concern over volume overloading this patient with end-stage renal disease (and a now- nonfunctioning dialysis catheter).

Which of the following would the initial hemodynamic profile for this patient most resemble?

	Cardiac Output L/min	Systemic Vascular Resistance mmHg	Wedge Pressure dynes-sec/cm5
A.	High	Low	Low
B.	Low	High	Low
C.	Low	High	High
D.	Low	High	Normal/Low

180.

A 16-year-old boy is brought to the ER by friends. The patient was at a party with his friends when he became confused and then unresponsive. On exam: BP 60/30 mmHg, P 140 bpm, T 97° F, O_2 saturation 88%. He has marked cyanosis of his extremities. He has marked cyanosis of his lips also.

Labs: Hb 14, HCT 42, WBC 1,000, ABG-pH 7.32, PO_2 46, PCO_2 44, Na 136, K 4.0, Cl 105, HCO_3 20.

The patient is placed on 100% O_2 by mask without improvement in his cyanosis.

Which of the following therapy should he receive?

A. Amyl nitrite
B. Bicarbonate drip
C. Narcan
D. Methylene blue
E. IV alcohol

ENDOCRINOLOGY

181.

A parent calls your office concerned that her child may have diabetes. The child is a 2-year-old female with a history of increased thirst, but no increased urine output. Her weight is stable and her appetite is normal. She is acting normal. Her grandmother has Type 2 diabetes and Mom used Grandma's meter to check her daughter's blood sugar, to find it was 150 mg/dL.

Which of the following is the most appropriate next step in managing this patient?

A. Admit to the hospital for diabetes education and management.
B. Give 2 units of insulin aspart (NovoLog®).
C. Reassure and educate about the diagnosis and presentation of diabetes.
D. Have her drink water, then check blood sugar in 2 hours on her grandmother's meter again.
E. Present to the clinic in the morning for an oral glucose tolerance test.

182.

A mom brings in her daughter for evaluation of a neck rash. Per mom, "I thought she did not take a bath for a few days. I have tried to scrub it off, but it will not disappear." On exam of the 13-year-old female, you notice a dark, velvety rash around her neck and axilla, and behind her knees.

Which of the following lab would most likely be elevated?

A. Cortisol
B. Insulin
C. Growth hormone
D. Cholesterol
E. Triglyceride

183.

A dad presents with his 14-year-old daughter for a routine physical exam. He wants to know if she should have any health screening labs done. She is Caucasian and normal weight. There is a family history of T2DM. She has normal menses. She denies any skin rashes. He is very worried about diabetes.

Which of the following do you recommend?

A. Screening for diabetes with a random glucose level
B. Screening for diabetes with a fasting glucose level
C. Screening for diabetes with an insulin level
D. Screening for diabetes with a hemoglobulin A1C
E. Not screening for diabetes

184.

A 15-year-old African-American male presents to the clinic with complaints of fatigue and increased thirst. His blood sugar was 250, with normal sodium and potassium, and with no evidence of acidosis or ketones. His morning fasting blood sugar was 180. You diagnose T2DM.

The parents ask about management.

Which of the following would be the most appropriate initial step in his management?

    A. Diet and exercise with repeat labs in 3 months
    B. Insulin therapy
    C. Sulfonylurea therapy
    D. TZD therapy

185.

You see a 13-year-old male in the clinic. You notice an increased waist circumference, a BMI > 95%, and a blood pressure greater than the 95th percentile for age and height. You diagnose metabolic syndrome.

Which of the following associated diseases do you need to counsel and screen for?

    A. Fatty liver
    B. Type 2 diabetes
    C. Cardiovascular disease
    D. Fatty liver, Type 2 diabetes, and cardiovascular disease
    E. Hypothyroidism

186.

The mother of a 7-year-old boy with T1DM calls the clinic because his morning blood sugars are always elevated. He is on 12 NPH and sliding scale insulin aspart (NovoLog®) in the morning, sliding scale insulin aspart at dinner, and 6 units of NPH at bedtime.

Which one of the following do you recommend?

    A. Increasing his evening NPH to 8 units
    B. Changing his NPH to glargine (Lantus®)
    C. Decreasing his evening NPH to 6 units
    D. Checking his blood sugar at 0300
    E. Changing his sliding scale at dinner

187.

A 4-year-old female presents to the ER with polyuria, polydipsia, and weight loss. Her initial labs at presentation are a pH of 7.1, BG of 560, and a HCO_3 of 9. She is diagnosed with DKA and sent to the PICU for management. She starts to complain of headache and becomes sleepy 10 hours into management. You diagnose cerebral edema.

Which one of the following is true concerning cerebral edema?

A. Treatment is with dexamethasone and hyperventilation.
B. Mortality is 50%.
C. Risk factors include new-onset IDDM and age < 5 years.
D. Risk factors include hyperkalemia at presentation.
E. This occurs in 10% of patients with DKA.

188.

A 14-year-old male with T1DM for 6 years presents for follow-up. He needs to have his annual labs done. He has had all appropriate screening done in the past during his usual checkups. Previous thyroid tests done yearly are normal, as are lipids done last year.

Which pair of the following tests and referrals needs to be done this year due to his diabetes being present for > 5 years?

A. Microalbuminuria and colonoscopy
B. Microalbuminuria and ophthalmology
C. Anti-TPO and ophthalmology
D. Anti-TPO and colonoscopy
E. Lipid profile and ophthalmology

189.

A 12-year-old male with IDDM awoke this morning with a BG of 450. He is on 25 units of insulin glargine (Lantus®) and an insulin/carb ratio of 1/15 with all meals. He has had URI symptoms and a low-grade fever for a few days. He has not had any emesis to date. You ask him to begin his sick-day regimen.

All of the following should be in his regimen except:

A. Monitor ketones with BG > 250.
B. Give insulin glargine every 3 hours according to his sliding scale.
C. Give promethazine if he develops emesis.
D. Drink at least 8 ounces of fluid an hour.
E. Eat at least 15 gm of carbs an hour.

190.

A 3-year-old female presents with a history of breast enlargement. She has no evidence of any androgen effects. You suspect premature thelarche.

Which of the following is the most appropriate evaluation for premature thelarche?

A. Bone age, DHEAS, estradiol
B. Bone age, estradiol, thyroid function tests, LH/FSH
C. Bone age, estradiol, LH/FSH
D. Bone age, beta-hCG, testosterone, 17-OHP
E. Bone age, LH/FSH, prolactin

191.

A 15-year-old asymptomatic African-American male with a BMI > 85%, a positive family history of Type 2 diabetes, and acanthosis nigricans has a fasting blood sugar of 110 mg/dL.

Which of the following is the best next step in determining if he has Type 2 diabetes?

A. Repeat a fasting blood sugar.
B. Check a HbA1c.
C. Perform a glucose tolerance test.
D. Check a fasting insulin level.
E. Check a random glucose level.

192.

A 13-year-old female presents to the hospital in diabetic ketoacidosis. This is her third admission for DKA this year. Her HbA1c is 13%.

Which of the following is the most likely reason for her multiple admissions for DKA?

A. Noncompliance with her diabetes management
B. Insulin resistance
C. Puberty hormones
D. Overeating
E. Insulin antibodies

193.

A 3-year-old female presents with a history of menstrual bleeding. On exam, she has Tanner stage 1 breast development and Tanner stage 1 pubic hair. The rest of her exam is normal except for a large café-au-lait spot on her chest.

Which of the following is the most likely reason for her menstrual bleeding?

A. McCune-Albright syndrome
B. Neurofibromatosis
C. Premature menarche
D. Precocious puberty
E. Tuberous sclerosis

194.

A 15-year-old boy presents for evaluation of pubertal delay. On exam, his pubic hair development is Tanner stage 1, and his testes are descended and are 3 cc in volume. He is otherwise healthy. On review of systems, he admits to having difficulty with his sense of smell. You suspect Kallmann syndrome.

Which of the following is the genetic defect associated with this syndrome?

A. Deletion q11–13 region of chromosome 15
B. Mutation of the *KAL* gene at Xp22.3, which results in a migration gene defect
C. Missense mutation in the gene coding for the alpha subunit of the stimulatory G protein
D. Deletion of chromosome 12q
E. Chromosomal abnormality with karyotype 47,XXY

195.

A 9-year-old boy presents for his routine physical exam. He continues to grow at the 5th percentile for height and weight.

Which one of the following tests will differentiate constitutional growth delay from genetic short stature?

A. IGF-1
B. IGF-BP3
C. Bone age
D. Growth hormone level
E. TSH

196.

A 16-year-old female presents with complaints of tremor, heat intolerance, and weight loss. She has a goiter on exam, and her resting heart rate is 120 beats/minute. You suspect hyperthyroidism.

Which of the following is the most appropriate initial workup to diagnose this disorder?

A. Free T4, TSH, thyroid ultrasound
B. Free T4, TSH, thyroglobulin, thyroid-stimulating immunoglobulin
C. T3, free T4, TSH, thyroid antibodies
D. Free T4, TSH, thyroid-stimulating immunoglobulin
E. Free T4, TSH, thyroid-stimulating immunoglobulin, thyroid ultrasound

197.

You are called by the state health department due to an abnormal newborn screen. Your patient is a 3-day-old male with a low T4 and a normal TSH. You call the patient in for an exam. This exam is normal—the baby is feeding well, is gaining weight, and has no clinical evidence of hypothyroidism on exam. On repeat labs, the baby's TSH remains normal. His T4 is low but his free T4 is normal.

Which one of the following additional tests must you order to make the diagnosis in this patient?

A. Total T3
B. Thyroglobulin
C. Thyroid antibodies
D. Thyroid-binding globulin
E. Thyroid

198.

A 16-month-old male presents for evaluation of bowed legs. He has been healthy. On exam, you notice his growth velocity to be poor—he has fallen to less than the 5th percentile in length. His father is short and also has bowed legs. Your evaluation includes a normal calcium level of 9.0 mg/dL but a low phosphorus level of 2.0 mg/dL (normal 3.2–6.3 mg/dL). You suspect hypophosphatemic rickets.

Of the following options, which is necessary to treat hypophosphatemic rickets?

    A. Vitamin D and calcium
    B. Phosphorus and vitamin D
    C. Phosphorus and calcium
    D. Phosphorus only
    E. Vitamin D only

199.

A 5-day-old, full-term baby presents to the ER with a hypocalcemic seizure. He was delivered at home. You do not have any records of his prenatal care or his birth history. This is his first seizure, according to his mom.

Which of the following is the most likely reason for his seizure?

    A. Infant of a diabetic mom
    B. IUGR
    C. Hypoparathyroidism
    D. Sepsis
    E. Birth asphyxia

200.

You are taking care of a 12-year-old female with T1DM. She was recently diagnosed with Addison disease. You suspect Type 2 autoimmune polyendocrinopathy.

Which one of the following is she most at risk for in this syndrome?

    A. Hypothyroidism
    B. Chronic mucocutaneous candidiasis
    C. Chronic active hepatitis
    D. Nail disease
    E. Hyperparathyroidism

201.

A 12-year-old boy with a history of significant behavioral problems and pervasive developmental disorder (PDD) takes several medications in an attempt to allow him to participate in class activities at his school. His parents present with concerns that he has developed a milky discharge from both breasts. He is otherwise well and in his normal state of health, which, from a physical standpoint, is excellent.

Which of the following medications is the most likely cause of this patient's symptoms?

A. Risperidone
B. Methylphenidate
C. Amphetamine and dextroamphetamine
D. Atomoxetine
E. Fluoxetine

202.

A 16-year-old male with a history of red-green color blindness is referred for delayed puberty. Soon after birth, he underwent repair of a cleft lip/palate. The tone of his voice confirms that it has not deepened. He has no facial hair and little increase in muscle bulk. Testicular volume is estimated at 4–5 mL.

Which of the following findings on physical examination is likely to be identified during additional evaluation of this patient?

A. Small, deformed pinna associated with preauricular pitting
B. Optic nerve coloboma
C. Port-wine facial nevus
D. Multiple café au lait spots associated with axillary freckling
E. Abnormal results during testing of the first cranial nerve

203.

A 16-year-old female presents with the complaint of excessive facial hair. This has continued to become more prominent during the previous several years. Her BMI is $> 99^{th}$ percentile. A preliminary diagnosis of polycystic ovary syndrome is established.

Which of the following laboratory findings would be most consistent with this syndrome?

A. Elevated free serum testosterone
B. Decreased serum levels of both LH and FSH
C. Elevated serum levels of FSH associated with an FSH:LH ratio of $> 2:1$
D. Elevated serum levels of estradiol, of at least 2x normal for the follicular phase of menses
E. Elevated serum levels of progesterone, of at least 2x normal for the luteal phase of menses

204.

A 17-year-old female returns for follow-up after starting oral contraceptive pills as treatment for polycystic ovary syndrome. She is frustrated by the lack of improvement in the appearance of excessive facial hair and acne and requests an alternative treatment.

Which of the following medications represents the most appropriate next step in the treatment of this patient?

A. A progestin-only oral contraceptive pill
B. Depot medroxyprogesterone (Depo-Provera®), 150 mg IM every 90 days
C. A once-daily long-acting insulin preparation
D. Hydrochlorothiazide
E. Spironolactone

205.

The mother of an 11-year-old girl presents with the concern that her daughter appears to have had a persistent vaginal discharge during the previous 2 months. On physical examination, she is in the 45th percentile for height and weight. Her breasts are enlarged without separation of areolar contour from the breast. Coarse, curly pubic hair extends over the mid-pubis. Moderate vaginal discharge is noted. Wet prep shows numerous epithelial cells.

Which of the following is the most appropriate next step in the treatment of this child?

A. Oral fluconazole
B. Single-dose therapy with oral metronidazole
C. Topical clotrimazole
D. Oral cefdinir
E. Reassurance that no additional treatment is indicated

206.

The parents of a 3-year-old girl present for a routinely scheduled health maintenance examination. Their only concern is a "small lump in her neck," present for the last several weeks and unchanged in size or location.

Which of the following findings suggests that the mass is due to a thyroglossal duct cyst?

A. A tender cyst-like mass lateral to the hyoid bone
B. A superficial mobile cyst-like mass just medial to the anterior cervical chain at the level of the thyroid cartilage
C. A nontender cyst-like mass in the lower left lobe of the thyroid gland
D. A firm, fixed, tender cyst-like mass just above the midline of the suprasternal notch
E. A midline cyst-like mass at the level of the hyoid bone, which moves upward with swallowing

207.

During a health maintenance visit, the parents of a 4-year-old boy mention that they were surprised their son had been unaware that his dog had been sprayed by a skunk several days earlier. They go on to say that he continued to play with and pet the dog despite the fact that the dog "smelled awful." Formal assessment of the first cranial nerve confirms an inability to smell.

Which of the following is most likely to be an associated finding in this patient?

A. Previous repair of a cleft lip/cleft palate
B. A seizure disorder
C. Blue sclera associated with generalized osteoporosis
D. Albinism
E. Multiple cavernous hemangiomas

208.

An 18-year-old college freshman presents for follow-up after he was found to have an LDL of 162 mg/dL and a triglyceride level of 240 mg/dL. He was initially evaluated because of a positive family history of early cardiac disease. He states that he "is careful about what he eats" but goes on to say that he has recently gained 15 pounds to "buff up for football." On physical exam, his blood pressure is 150/105 mmHg.

Assuming that his laboratory and clinical findings are due to the use of anabolic steroids, which of the following findings is most likely to be identified in this patient?

A. Increased testicular size
B. Gynecomastia
C. A thyroid nodule
D. Increased intraocular pressure
E. Pseudotumor cerebri

209.

During a scheduled health maintenance exam, a 10-month-old girl is noted to have bilateral asymmetric breast development. Her parents first noticed breast development about 6 weeks prior to presentation and believe that her breasts continue to increase in size. On physical examination, she is at the 30th percentile for both height and weight; her head circumference is at the 45th percentile. Both breasts are enlarged, the left more than the right. There is no evidence of galactorrhea, pubic hair, or thickening of the vaginal mucosa.

Which of the following is the most appropriate next step in the evaluation of this patient?

A. Obtain levels of thyroid-stimulating hormone and thyroxine.
B. Obtain a chromosome analysis.
C. Obtain levels of serum testosterone and androstenedione.
D. Obtain levels of serum 17-beta-estradiol.
E. Reevaluate the patient in 3–6 months.

210.

A 17-year-old competitive figure skater presents with a 5-month history of amenorrhea. Menarche was at 14 years of age. She denies sexual activity and chronic illness and takes no daily medications. She competes throughout the year and practices each morning for 3 hours before going to school. She is at the 5th percentile for weight and the 60th percentile for height. Her physical exam is unremarkable. Urine pregnancy test is negative.

Which of the following complications is most likely to occur in this patient?

A. Thromboembolism
B. Altered lipid metabolism with a disproportionate increase in low-density lipoproteins
C. Loss of bone mineral density
D. Fatty liver disease (steatorrheic hepatosis)
E. Insulin-dependent diabetes mellitus

211.

A 19-year-old female presents after "missing her last three periods." Menarche occurred at 12 years of age. She reports that she had regular menstrual periods until 16 years of age. Since that time, she has experienced cyclical abdominal pain, although her menses are irregular and less frequent. She has had two miscarriages—one at 17 years of age and the second 7 months prior to presentation. Both occurred at approximately 14-weeks gestation and required curettage to control excessive bleeding. A urine pregnancy test is negative. No specific abnormalities are identified on pelvic examination.

Which of the following is the most likely cause of secondary amenorrhea in this patient?

A. Tubo-ovarian abscess
B. Intrauterine adhesions
C. Endometriosis
D. Premature ovarian failure
E. Polycystic ovary syndrome

212.

A 5-year-old male presents to your clinic for a routine physical exam. His exam is normal except for evidence of some pubic hair. His testes are 3 cc and are descended bilaterally. On further questioning, his mom states she has been giving him some deodorant for his body odor. You suspect premature adrenarche but need to rule out more serious diseases.

Which of the following should you include in your initial workup?

A. Testosterone, FSH/LH, bone age, DHEAS, TFTs
B. Testosterone, DHEAS, androstenedione, bone age, 17-OHP
C. Prolactin, testosterone, bone age, TFTs
D. FSH/LH, testosterone, cortisol, bone age
E. Testosterone, androstenedione, cortisol, TFTs, bone age

213.

An 8-year-old boy presents for a routine physical. On exam, he has Tanner 2 pubic hair and 5 cc bilaterally descended testes.

Which of the following is the most appropriate test to order now?

A. Testicular ultrasound
B. Brain and sella MRI
C. Bone age
D. Adrenal CT
E. Testosterone level

214.

A 2-year-old female presents with short stature and a web neck. You suspect Turner or Noonan syndrome.

Which of the following would help make the diagnosis of Noonan syndrome in this patient?

A. Pulmonary stenosis and mental retardation
B. Aortic insufficiency and hearing deficiency
C. Renal pathology and cubitus valgus
D. Wilms tumor
E. Short fourth metacarpal

215.

You are seeing a 15-year-old male with obesity, hypogonadism, and mental retardation. On review of his chart, you see he has been diagnosed with retinitis pigmentosa.

Which of the following disorders does this patient most likely have?

A. Prader-Willi syndrome
B. Klinefelter syndrome
C. Kallmann syndrome
D. Laurence-Moon-Biedel/Bardet-Biedel syndrome
E. Sertoli-cell-only syndrome

216.

You are seeing a 15-year-old male in the clinic. The parents are concerned with his size. He is currently at the 5th percentile for height and weight—and has been growing at this percentile for years. His midparental height is 72 inches. He has an excellent appetite and is very active after school. His exam is normal except for Tanner stage 2 pubic hair and 5 cc testes. His bone age is 13 years.

Which of the following should you recommend?

A. Testosterone level
B. FSH/LH
C. Testicular ultrasound
D. Dietary consult
E. Reassurance and follow-up exam in 6 months

217.

A 16-year-old male presents to your clinic for a sports physical for football. He has no complaints at presentation. His history reveals some learning difficulties in school. On exam, you notice bilateral gynecomastia. His genital exam is remarkable for Tanner 4 pubic hair and 8 cc testes.

Which one of the following tests should you order to make his diagnosis?

A. A drug screen for anabolic steroids
B. Prolactin
C. Chromosomes
D. Estradiol
E. Testosterone

218.

A female patient presents to your clinic with short stature. Her weight's percentile is greater than that of her height. Her fingers and toes appear short. You notice several members of her family with a similar appearance. Her labs return with calcium of 6.8 (low), phosphorus of 7.0 (high), and PTH of 100 (elevated).

Which of the following is the most likely diagnosis?

A. Hypoparathyroidism
B. Pseudohypoparathyroidism
C. Pseudopseudohypoparathyroidism
D. Vitamin D–deficient rickets
E. Hypophosphatemic rickets

219.

You are called to the nursery to see a 2-day-old male with recurrent hypoglycemia. His exam is normal except for a penile length of 1.8 cm.

Which of the following is most likely?

A. Growth hormone deficiency
B. Testosterone deficiency
C. XX karyotype
D. Hypothyroidism
E. Androgen insensitivity syndrome

220.

Which one of the following is <u>not</u> an FDA-approved use for growth hormone therapy?

A. Growth hormone deficiency
B. Turner syndrome
C. Prader-Willi syndrome
D. Down syndrome
E. Renal osteodystrophy

221.

A baby in the nursery has macroglossia, hypoglycemia, and hepatosplenomegaly. You suspect Beckwith-Wiedemann syndrome.

Children with Beckwith-Wiedemann syndrome are most at risk for developing which of the following?

A. Wilms tumor
B. Ewing sarcoma
C. Pheochromocytoma
D. Medulloblastoma
E. Leukemia

222.

A 3-year-old female presents to the ER with seizures due to hypoglycemia. She had been well until yesterday, when she started to have acute gastrointestinal symptoms. She has not eaten well since yesterday morning. Her blood sugar at presentation is 35 ng/dL.

Which one of the following lab test combinations are most needed to help determine the etiology of her hypoglycemia?

A. TSH, fT4, cortisol, glucose, growth hormone
B. Cortisol, glucose, growth hormone, insulin, ketones
C. Cortisol, glucose, C-peptide, insulin, pro insulin
D. Glucose, cortisol, growth hormone, ketones, C-peptide
E. TSH, fT4, insulin, glucose, growth hormone

223.

You receive a call from the state lab stating that one of your patients has a positive result for congenital adrenal hyperplasia (CAH) on his newborn screening. His result for CAH was 641 nanograms/mL (normal for his birth weight of 8 lb 7 oz is < 55 nanograms/mL). You saw him at 5 days of age for a well check, at which time his weight was 7 lb, 7 oz. He was alert and looked fine, except he was jaundiced with a bilirubin of 17.8. Both testicles were down. You continued to follow his bilirubin level and weight over the next several days. At 8 days of age, his weight was 7 lb, 4 oz with a bilirubin level of 18.2. You get the call from the lab the following day, when the infant is 9 days old.

Which one of the following labs would be most important to order right away?

A. 17-alpha-hydroxyprogesterone (17-OHP) and electrolytes.
B. 17-OHP only.
C. Estrone level.
D. Estradiol level.
E. No need to order other tests at this time. You can wait for the 2nd newborn screening results at 2 weeks of age.

224.

You are seeing a 3-year-old female for the first time for short stature. Mother reports she has always been short. She has had numerous ear infections and was diagnosed as an infant with a bicuspid aortic valve.

On physical examination, she is well below the 5th percentile for height. She has a short neck, low hairline, high-arched palate, protruding ears, and short metacarpals.

Which of the following is the most likely diagnosis?

A. Growth hormone deficiency
B. Constitutional delay
C. Cushing syndrome
D. Turner syndrome
E. Laron syndrome

225.

A 14-year-old male presents to your clinic with a "swollen left nipple" for 2 weeks. Occasionally, it is tender. No discharge. No redness or fever. He has had no chronic illnesses.

On physical examination, he appears healthy. He has a 2 cm, firm, freely movable, subareolar mass on the left breast that is mildly tender. No redness or discharge. No mass palpated in the right breast.

Which of the following is the most likely diagnosis?

A. Breast cancer
B. Subareolar abscess
C. Rhabdomyosarcoma
D. Physiologic pubertal gynecomastia
E. Liposarcoma

226.

Which of the following is most useful in determining the bone age of a child?

A. Width-length ratios of certain bones as compared to known standards
B. Width of the skull
C. Width of the bones of the hands
D. Radiodensity of vertebrae as compared to known standards
E. The presence or absence of specific ossification centers as compared to known standards

227.

Which one of the following best represents when maximal growth in muscle mass occurs?

A. Just before puberty begins
B. After the maximal growth in height
C. After puberty is done
D. At age 40 when one starts lifting weights
E. Paralleling the maximal growth in height

228.

Which one of the following best indicates Tanner stage 3 of sexual development in a girl?

A. Acne
B. Menarche
C. Breast and papilla elevated as a small mound
D. Darkly pigmented, slightly curly pubic hair
E. Light pubic hair

229.

Which one of the following statements about familial short stature is true?

A. Growth retardation develops in later childhood.
B. Ultimate height is average.
C. The onset of puberty is delayed.
D. The shape of the growth curve is abnormally concave.
E. The bone age is usually normal or only slightly delayed.

230.

Which one of the following is true in children with isolated growth hormone deficiency?

A. They show slowing of growth velocity but remain on the growth curve.
B. They show slowing of growth velocity and fall off the normal growth curve.
C. They have a normal bone age.
D. They have associated mild hypothyroidism.
E. They have associated brain tumors.

231.

A 16-year-old female presents with delayed puberty. She has no other endocrine abnormality in her workup.

Which of the following is likely to be true?

A. She will likely be normal height and weight.
B. She will be short and obese.
C. She will be short and have proportionate weight.
D. She will be very tall and be obese.
E. She will be very tall and play basketball for a pro basketball team and makes lots of money, and you will able to sit in the front row because you are her doctor.

232.

Which of the following is the commonest time frame for ovulation to begin in an adolescent girl?

A. Following menarche by 1 to 2 months
B. Following menarche by 12 to 24 months
C. At the same time as menarche
D. Preceding menarche by 1 to 2 months
E. Preceding menarche by 12 to 24 months

233.

Which one of the following is true in an adolescent girl regarding the timing of menarche?

A. It precedes the growth spurt.
B. It occurs with Tanner stage 3.
C. It occurs 2 years after Tanner stage 5.
D. It usually occurs at the same time as Tanner stages 4 to 5.
E. It occurs with Tanner stage 2.

234.

A 6-year-old child (at the 50th percentile for height) suddenly stops growing and, by age 10, is off the growth curve (< 5th percentile). He essentially has not grown since age 7.

Which of the following is the most likely etiology?

A.   Craniopharyngioma
B.   Congenital hypothyroidism
C.   Normal variant
D.   Constitutional growth delay
E.   Androgen excess

ENT / OPHTHALMOLOGY / ORTHOPEDICS

235.

A 3-year-old boy awakens from his sleep complaining of pain when attempting to move his neck. His mother also reports that he has been drooling and has had difficulty swallowing for the last 24 hours. On physical examination his temperature is 103.1° F. He has some intermittent stridor and holds his neck in a hyperextended position. There is what appears to be a puncture wound on his soft palate.

Which of the following is likely to be identified upon further evaluation of this patient?

    A. A swollen "cherry red" epiglottis on direct laryngoscopy in the operating room
    B. Increased width of the soft tissues in the retropharyngeal space on lateral roentgenogram
    C. Asymmetric enlargement of one tonsil with deviation of the uvula and soft palate edema
    D. Extensive dental carries associated with gingival hyperplasia and bleeding
    E. A foreign body lodged in the pharynx distal to the tonsillar tissue

236.

A 9-year-old boy presents with a 24-hour history of sore throat, malaise, and decreased appetite. He attends third grade, where several other classmates have similar symptoms. His parents are concerned that "strep throat might be going around" in his classroom. A rapid strep test (RST) is negative.

Which of the following is most likely to be associated with viral pharyngitis as compared to group A streptococcal (GAS) disease?

    A. Absence of nasal discharge and cough
    B. Tender anterior cervical lymphadenopathy
    C. Erythematous conjunctiva associated with discharge and photophobia
    D. A fine macular papular rash on the trunk and groin
    E. Soft palate petechiae

237.

A 4-year-old child with trisomy 21 and a history of recurrent otitis media presents complaining of left ear pain. He has twice undergone tympanostomy tube placement, most recently 11 months ago. His left tympanic membrane is erythematous and full. In addition, a discrete, grayish-white, somewhat rounded, opaque structure is identified on the superior portion of the tympanic membrane.

Which of the following is the most likely cause of this finding?

    A. A cholesteatoma
    B. A partially extruded tympanostomy tube
    C. A hardened piece of cerumen
    D. Tympanosclerosis
    E. A retraction pocket due to negative pressure within the middle ear cavity

238.

The parents of a 2-year-old girl present with the concern that their daughter's "pink eye is suddenly much worse." Two days prior to presentation they started to administer a topical antibiotic in her right eye that was "left over" from a prior infection. In addition, her parents report that she has had a cough and nasal discharge during the preceding week. Her past medical history is otherwise negative, and her immunizations are up-to-date. Upon arrival, her temperature is 102.9° F. She appears quite ill with significant edema, which is both tender and warm to palpation, of the upper and lower lids and surrounding tissue of the right eye. There is also clear evidence of proptosis of the right eye.

Which of the following represents the most likely finding upon further evaluation of this patient?

A. Positive blood culture for *Haemophilus influenzae* type b
B. Heavy growth of *Neisseria meningitides* following culture of conjunctival discharge
C. Opacification of the ethmoid sinuses on CT scan
D. Papilledema on examination of the right fundus
E. Evidence of herpetic (dendritic) keratitis on slit lamp examination of the right eye

239.

The parents of a 2-year-old boy present with the concern that their son is "having trouble breathing." He has a 2-day history of cough, nasal discharge, and decreased appetite. On physical examination his temperature is 101.1° F, respiratory rate is 38. He appears uncomfortable but remains calm when sitting in his mother's lap. When offered, he readily accepts and drinks a glass of water. Audible inspiratory stridor is noted, which worsens when he is examined.

Which of the following x-ray findings is most likely to be identified during further evaluation of this patient?

A. Right middle lobe consolidation
B. Subglottic narrowing of the tracheal air column
C. Enlarged epiglottis protruding from the anterior wall of the hypopharynx
D. Foreign body in the right main stem bronchus
E. Widening of the retropharyngeal soft tissue (prevertebral space) associated with an air-fluid level

240.

A 6-week-old boy presents as jaundiced during a scheduled well-child examination. He appears lethargic and is reported to feed poorly. He is 1 pound above birth weight. Additional findings on physical examination include nystagmus and micropenis. Results of laboratory testing reveal a glucose of 38 mg/dL and an indirect bilirubin of 11 mg/dL.

Which of the following findings is most likely to be identified during additional evaluation of this patient?

A. Biliary atresia
B. Agenesis of the septum pellucidum
C. Bilateral cataracts
D. Positive PCR for herpes virus on examination of CSF
E. Hydronephrosis associated with posterior urethral valves

241.

During a routinely scheduled health maintenance exam, a 3-year-old boy with a history of recurrent otitis media is noted to have a discrete, smooth, grayish-white, rounded, opaque lesion in the superior portion of the right tympanic membrane.

Based upon the results of this patient's findings, which of the following is the most appropriate next step in the treatment of this patient?

A. Begin treatment with both oral amoxicillin and ofloxacin otic drops.
B. Observation only with recheck in 6 months.
C. Begin treatment with ofloxacin otic drops.
D. Refer for surgical excision only if there is evidence of hearing loss and/or language delay.
E. Refer for surgical excision.

242.

A 2-week-old infant is noted to have continued difficulty with feeding. He latches well to his mother's breast but soon after beginning to feed, he coughs and begins choking. In addition, his cry is weak and at times indiscernible. The infant is taken to the operating room, where direct laryngoscopy reveals unilateral vocal fold paralysis.

Which of the following is associated with an increased risk of vocal cord paralysis?

A. Difficult breech delivery
B. Thyroglossal duct cyst
C. Cystic hygroma
D. Cleft lip/cleft palate
E. Tracheoesophageal fistula

243.

A 19-month-old boy presents with a 1-day history of increased temperature, decreased appetite and fussiness. His parents also report that he "acts like he has a sore throat," with crying and drooling when attempting to feed. On physical examination his temperature is 104.9° F. He is irritable, but will become calm when allowed to sit in his mother's lap. There are scattered discrete vesicles surrounded by erythema, some of which have ulcerated, on the anterior tonsillar pillars, uvula, and posterior pharyngeal wall.

Which of the following is the most likely cause of these clinical findings?

A. Group A coxsackievirus
B. *Haemophilus influenzae* type b
C. Parainfluenza virus Type 2
D. Herpes virus Type 1
E. Adenovirus Type 4

244.

An 11-year-old girl presents with a history of sore throat, difficulty swallowing, and increased temperature. On physical examination, both tonsils are enlarged and covered with exudate. A rapid streptococcal test is positive.

Which of the following disorders is sometimes worsened by an intercurrent infection caused by group A streptococcus?

A. Visual and auditory hallucinations
B. Obsessive-compulsive behaviors
C. Oppositional-defiant behaviors
D. Depression
E. Narcolepsy

245.

An 11-year-old boy presents with a 2-week history of worsening pain in the proximal portion of his right femur. It has progressed to the point where it has awakened him from his sleep several times during the preceding week. During examination, he complains of significant pain upon palpation. He is also noted to have limited range of motion and decreased strength in the right lower extremity. An x-ray shows a round metaphyseal lucency surrounded by sclerotic bone.

Which of the following is the most appropriate next step in the treatment of this patient?

A. Trial of salicylate therapy
B. Trial of non-steroidal antiinflammatory therapy
C. Aspiration and biopsy of the lesion under fluoroscopy
D. Bone marrow aspiration
E. Open biopsy under general anesthesia

246.

A 15-year-old boy presents for a preparticipation sports physical. Over the previous several years he has become an accomplished tennis player, often practicing 2–3 hours/day.

Which of the following orthopedic problems is this patient at greatest risk of developing as he continues to practice and compete?

A. Medial epicondylitis
B. Avulsion of a portion of the tibial tubercle
C. Slipped capital femoral epiphysis
D. Subluxation of the patella
E. Lateral epicondylitis

247.

A 15-year-old boy presents complaining of knee pain that continues to interfere with his athletic activities. His left knee has bothered him "off and on" for several months. He goes on to state that the pain increases with activity and when he "stretches his legs during warm-ups." His knee will also "sometimes lock up," making it impossible for him to continue activity. On examination of the left knee, there is soft tissue swelling and joint line tenderness. During internal rotation of the tibia with the knee flexed to 90°, he complains of increased pain as the knee is slowly extended. Full extension of the knee is limited.

Which of the following findings is likely to be identified on a plain radiograph during further evaluation?

  A. A bony fragment in the medial condyle of the femur
  B. Fragmentation at the anterior tibial tubercle
  C. A lucent fracture line across the distal third of the patella
  D. Dislocation of the patella lateral to the femoral grove
  E. A small avulsion fragment from the inferior pole of the patella

248.

A 14-year-old boy complains of worsening left knee pain, which he first noticed 6 weeks prior to presentation. Although the pain did not initially interfere with activity, his parents have recently noticed that he sometimes will limp, especially when running or climbing stairs. Tenderness and soft-tissue prominence of the tibial tubercle is noted on physical examination. He complains of pain when the knee is extended against resistance and with squatting.

Which of the following is the most likely cause of these symptoms?

  A. Rupture of the anterior cruciate ligament
  B. Rupture of both the anterior and posterior cruciate ligaments
  C. Inflammation of the prepatellar bursa
  D. Inflammation of the connective tissue of the iliotibial band
  E. Avulsion causing separation of the proximal patellar tendon from its bony insertion

249.

A 4-year-old boy has refused to walk since awakening from a nap. His parents are not aware of any recent injury. He has been less active and more irritable over the last several days and has had an intermittent low-grade fever and complained of back pain. On physical examination his temperature is 100.9° F. His mobility is restricted, and he resists all attempts to encourage him to walk. There is localized tenderness over the T3-T4 area with associated paraspinal muscle spasm. Laboratory evaluation includes a WBC of 9,000 cells and an ESR of 95 mm/hr.

Which of the following is most likely to be identified upon further evaluation of this patient?

  A. Narrowing of the intervertebral disk space on MRI
  B. Positive blood culture for viridans streptococci
  C. Bone scan showing decreased perfusion to the femoral head
  D. A unilateral defect (separation) in the vertebral pars interarticularis
  E. Anterior wedging of 5 to 8 degrees in three adjacent vertebral bodies

250.

A 9-year-old female presents to your office with a 2-day history of sore throat, fever, and dysphagia. Her best friend was diagnosed with strep throat last week. She's had no vomiting or diarrhea but has had occasional headache and stomachache. She is allergic to amoxicillin but otherwise is very healthy.

Examination: T 101.9°   HR 100   RR 30   BP 105/69

She is alert but uncomfortable with trismus.
Oropharynx is red with pus, uvula swollen, slightly deviated to right, left tonsil is larger than the right.
Neck with swollen anterior cervical lymph nodes

The rest of exam is normal.

LABORATORY: Rapid strep test is positive.

Which of the following is the best next course of action?

    A. Send the patient home on amoxicillin.
    B. Send the patient home on erythromycin.
    C. Get a monospot and EBV titers and send patient home.
    D. Immediate consultation with ENT.
    E. Send patient home on antibiotics but add steroids to help with the swelling.

251.

You diagnose a 10-year-old boy with *Streptococcus pyogenes* pharyngitis. He requests an oral antibiotic instead of a "shot." You prescribe penicillin V-K 250 mg PO q 6 hours. His mother asks when he can return to school.

Which of the following represents when he could have safely returned to school, if he had received an IM injection of penicillin?

    A. 24 hours after his IM injection
    B. 48 hours after his IM injection
    C. 5 days after his IM injection
    D. Same day if he had received an IM injection
    E. 72 hours after his IM injection

252.

A 15-year-old male presents with a history of fever and sore throat associated with a pruritic rash. On physical examination you note pharyngeal exudates, cervical lymphadenopathy, and a maculopapular rash. The rash began on the extensor surfaces of the distal extremities and spread centripetally to the chest and back. It spares his face, palms, and soles.

A rapid strep test is negative as well as a monospot test. Cultures are sent for *Streptococcus pyogenes*.

Throat cultures return negative except for a Gram-positive rod that is growing only on blood-enriched media.

Which of the following is the most likely organism?

A. *Arcanobacterium haemolyticum*
B. *Streptococcus pyogenes*
C. Streptococcus Group C
D. *Bacillus anthracis*
E. *Corynebacterium diphtheriae*

253.

A 4-year-old boy presents with a swollen left cervical lymph node in the anterior chain just below the mandible. No cats are in the house, and his mother does not know of any animals that he has been around. He goes to daycare. He is begun on cephalexin and does not improve. He has low-grade temperatures, and the swelling continues to increase in size. It is now tender and erythematous. He does not have any other nodes. It has been 2 weeks since he was started on cephalexin, and in the last week he was begun on amoxicillin/clavulanate without improvement.

Which of the following is the most likely etiology of his condition?

A. Lymphoma
B. Leukemia
C. *Mycobacterium avium-intracellulare*
D. *Mycobacterium marinum*
E. Methicillin-resistant *Staphylococcus aureus*

254.

Which of the following is <u>not</u> true with regards to tympanometry?

A. Sensorineural hearing loss can be associated with a normal tympanogram.
B. Tympanometry can measure hearing sensitivity.
C. A child with normal hearing may have an abnormal tympanogram.
D. A "flat line" on tympanogram is associated with middle ear fluid.
E. A "low amplitude" tympanogram is associated with middle ear fluid.

255.

Which of the following ages is "conventional pure tone" audiometry screening first appropriate?

A. Infants less than 6 months of age
B. Newborns
C. 6 months to 2 years
D. School age children
E. Adolescents

256.

A 5-month-old graduate of the neonatal nursery presents for routine follow-up. He is a former 26-week gestation neonate. Brainstem-evoked auditory potential-auditory brainstem response (ABR) testing shows sensorineural hearing loss.

Which of the following is most likely responsible for these findings?

A. Perforated tympanic membrane
B. Tympanosclerosis
C. Chronic otitis media with effusion
D. Administration of aminoglycoside while in the neonatal intensive care unit
E. Cholesteatoma

257.

A 10-year-old boy comes in with acute ataxia and decreased ability to hear. He was at school and suddenly felt like he was going to fall down. His gait is wide spaced so he did not fall. Additionally, at approximately the same time he noted that he could not hear as well and felt a "fullness" in his ears.

Which of the following is the most likely diagnosis?

A. Perilymph fistula
B. Ménière's disease
C. Acute otitis media
D. Cerebellar brain tumor
E. Mastoiditis

258.

Bridget McDonald is a 3-year-old girl who is brought in by her mother. The child has complained of "ear hurt" for 1 day. She has no prior history of otitis media. She is afebrile.

When you attempt to examine her ear, she scampers to the other side of the room and says "ear hurt." After some persuasion and help from her mother, you are able to look at her ear. You note that it is **very** painful with movement of the pinna, but there is no erythema or warmth to it. Additionally, you now note a purulent discharge from the ear canal.

Which of the following is the most likely diagnosis?

A. Acute otitis media
B. Chronic otitis media
C. Foreign body in ear
D. Mastoiditis
E. Perilymph fistula

259.

A 16-year-old is brought in by his mother for recurrent nose bleeds. She reports that lately he seems to have nosebleeds all of the time. He is always rubbing his hand on his nose and needing extra tissues that he keeps in his pockets.

He does not have fever and does not complain of colds. On physical examination you note inflamed nasal turbinates and a perforation of his nasal septum. A nasal smear shows no eosinophils.

Which of the following should you evaluate for first?

A. Chronic rhinitis
B. Sinusitis
C. Dry air
D. Seasonal allergic rhinitis
E. Cocaine abuse

260.

Morgan Freed is a 5-year-old child who **loves** popsicles. Today while his mother was cleaning, he managed to get into the freezer and eat 10 popsicles in a period of 1 hour. He now has tender red nodules on his cheeks. He is afebrile and still has good oral intake (not for popsicles though!). The cheeks have full thickness erythema about a quarter in diameter, and the areas are firm-like nodules.

Which of the following is the most likely etiology?

A. Herpes simplex stimulated by the cold
B. Varicella zoster stimulated by the cold
C. Cold-induced cold abscesses (or popsicle panniculitis)
D. Oropharyngeal anaerobes stimulated by the cold
E. *Arcanobacterium haemolyticum* stimulated by the cold

261.

The mother of a 2-week-old baby calls stating her baby's eye is tearing excessively. At birth, the examining pediatrician informed the mother that the baby had nasolacrimal duct occlusion. The tearing has become worse, and the mother is more worried.

Which of the following is the most appropriate next step?

A. Ask the mother to bring the baby in for examination.
B. Reassure the mother that 90% of these cases resolve by the first year of life.
C. Advise gentle massage daily over the nasolacrimal duct.
D. Refer to an ophthalmologist.
E. Apply topical antibiotic eye drops.

262.

The mother of a 2-week-old baby calls stating her baby's eye is tearing excessively. At birth, the examining pediatrician informed the mother that the baby had nasolacrimal duct occlusion. The mother "walks in" to your office on Friday afternoon at 4:45, very anxious and upset that something is wrong with the baby. On physical examination, the baby's left eye is tearing excessively. You notice that the cornea of the left eye is slightly enlarged when compared with the cornea of the right eye. The baby is extremely uncooperative with ophthalmoscopic examination of the left eye, and so you are unable to elicit the red reflex. She also seems to be squinting to some extent.

Which of the following is most appropriate?

    A. Reassure the mother that 90% of these cases self resolve by the first year of life.
    B. Advise gentle massage over the nasolacrimal duct daily.
    C. Refer for immediate evaluation by an ophthalmologist.
    D. Refer to ophthalmologist for the next available appointment—about 6 weeks.
    E. Ask the mother to return with her baby next week because you are ready to go home.

263.

A 13-year-old boy is brought into the emergency room with a dramatic decrease in his visual acuity. He reports he was fine until yesterday when he thinks a metal sliver went into his eye while in shop class. He was trying to pry open a lock with a wrench and metal screwdriver when he had severe pain in his eye after one of his attempts. He does not remember seeing anything come into his eye. He tried washing his eye out, but the pain has persisted.

PHYSICAL EXAMINATION:
    Vital signs are normal
    Right eye: Normal
    Left eye: Severely erythematous with severe chemosis
    Slit lamp: Severe corneal deterioration with a ring abscess
                 Both chambers are full of debris and cells

    Plain X-ray: Shows a foreign body in the left eye

Which of the following is the most likely pathogen?

    A. *Bacillus cereus*
    B. *Acanthamoeba*
    C. *Bartonella henselae*
    D. *Staphylococcus epidermidis*
    E. *Streptococcus oralis*

264.

Which of the following statements is <u>not</u> true about strabismus?

A. Untreated strabismus leads to monocular visual loss.
B. Strabismic amblyopia is rarely treatable after 6 years of age.
C. The most effective treatment is occlusion of the "fixing" eye with a patch.
D. Strabismus is any malalignment of the 2 eyes so that the visual axes are not oriented on the same target in space.
E. Exotropia is more common than esotropia.

265.

Which of the following is true?

A. Myopia is common in early term infants.
B. Myopia refers to farsightedness.
C. Hyperopia usually requires spectacle correction if mild.
D. Contact lenses are not useful in children.
E. The majority of children with significant refractory errors have no complaints whatsoever.

266.

A 5-year-old boy is brought in by his mother because he keeps running into doors. On visual field testing he is unable to distinguish objects brought laterally toward the midline, encompassing nearly 1/2 of the visual field of each eye.

Which of the following lesions is most likely to account for his findings?

A. Open-angle glaucoma
B. Closed-angle glaucoma
C. Multiple sclerosis
D. Craniopharyngioma
E. Occipital tumor

267.

A 17-year-old girl is being evaluated for anisocoria. Her left pupil is small and round compared with the right pupil in room light. When you place her in a darkened room, this difference is increased. The left pupil responds briskly to light, constricts with pilocarpine administration, and dilates with atropine. Minimal dilatation is produced by 4% cocaine.

Which of the following is the most likely location for her lesion?

  A. Left sympathetic chain
  B. Left optic nerve
  C. Left iris
  D. Left third nerve
  E. Right occipital lobe

268.

On routine physical examination, a newborn infant is found to have photophobia (Wow, isn't that hard to assess in a newborn? Almost like figuring out if a cow has mad-cow disease—but I guess that goes more in the ID section), epiphora, blepharospasm, and enlarged and cloudy corneas.

Which of the following is most likely the cause of these findings?

  A. Galactosemia
  B. Congenital rubella
  C. Intraocular hemorrhages
  D. Congenital glaucoma
  E. Congenital cataracts

269.

Which of the following would you be worried about if a premature infant was exposed to an arterial PaO_2 greater than 100 mmHg for a prolonged period of time?

  A. Kernicterus
  B. Getting "high"
  C. Brain shrinkage
  D. Retinopathy of prematurity
  E. Corneal abrasions

270.

Which of the following is <u>not</u> true regarding Brushfield spots?

  A. They occur in Down syndrome children.
  B. They occur especially in babies with blue eyes.
  C. They are tiny white spots.
  D. They form a ring in the mid-zone of the iris.
  E. They are always abnormal.

271.

A 2-year-old boy presents to your office for a well child exam. The mother is worried because the child's right foot appears to be rotated internally when the child walks. The child has otherwise been healthy. There were no complications of pregnancy or delivery. His gross and fine motor development have been normal. On exam, you notice the same "intoeing" of the right foot. When sitting and dangling his legs, the lateral malleolus is slightly anterior to the medial malleolus of the affected leg.

Which of the following do you recommend to the mother?

A. Immediate orthopedic referral
B. Referral to an orthopedic surgeon at the next available appointment
C. Serial leg casting
D. Braces which will hold the leg in external rotation, to be worn while sleeping
E. No intervention—the problem will resolve itself with time

272.

A child returns to your office when he is 5 years old. When the child was 2 years old, the mother was worried because the child's right foot appeared to be rotated internally when the child walked. At that time you noticed the same "intoeing" of the right foot. When sitting and dangling his legs, the lateral malleolus was slightly anterior to the medial malleolus of the affected leg. At that time you recommended no intervention and informed the mother that the problem would resolve itself with time. The mother now complains that the same problem has recurred—he intoes with his right foot while walking. When the child is standing, you notice that the right patella points inward. With the child in the prone position, you are able to achieve 90-degree internal rotation of the right femur and only 45-degree internal rotation of the left femur. There are no other deformities. The child continues to develop normally.

Which of the following do you recommend to the mother?

A. Immediate orthopedic referral
B. Referral to an orthopedic surgeon at the next available appointment
C. Serial leg casting
D. Braces to hold the leg in external rotation
E. No intervention—the problem will resolve itself

273.

A 6-year-old Caucasian male presents with a 4-week history of right knee pain. He denies trauma to that leg. The pain has been getting progressively worse so that he now limps. There has been no fever. 1 year ago, he was diagnosed with nephrotic syndrome from minimal change disease. He was treated conventionally with good response. Otherwise, he has been healthy and developing normally. On physical examination, his height and weight are in the 10th percentile as they have been since 2 months of age. There is no obvious deformity, swelling, erythema, or bruising of the affected hip, knee, or leg. He is holding the affected leg in external rotation at the hip joint. He has a positive Trendelenburg's sign when balancing his weight on the affected leg. Hip x-ray reveals joint space widening on the affected side. WBC and ESR are normal.

Which of the following is the most likely diagnosis?

A. Legg-Calve-Perthes disease, or avascular necrosis of the femoral head
B. Slipped capital femoral epiphysis
C. Transient synovitis
D. Septic arthritis
E. Growing pains

274.

The mother of a 4-year-old brings the child in with acute arm pain. The child was playing on the playground at school. He was on top of the slide and started to slide down. Another child grabbed his hand and tried to pull him back up. The child turned and shrieked in pain. Frightened, the other child let go and the first child was dropped to the ground. The child has since refused to move his arm. On physical examination, there is no swelling of the arm. There is point tenderness over the supracondylar region. The child is holding the arm against his abdomen.

Which of the following is the best next step in this patient?

A. Supination followed by flexion of the arm
B. Immobilization
C. Immediate orthopedic referral
D. Immediate orthopedic referral followed by emergency surgery
E. X-ray of the elbow

275.

You are seeing a 13-year-old male for bilateral knee pain—actually the pain is just below his knees. He denies any trauma to his legs. He is currently playing soccer and just started track 2 weeks ago. He first noticed the pain 1 week ago, and it is now occurring every time he runs. The pain goes away when he rests.

He has been very healthy. Family history is non-contributory.
On physical examination, both knees and legs look normal. No swelling. Tenderness to palpation is elicited over the tibial tubercle bilaterally. The tenderness is also elicited by knee extension against resistance.

Which of the following is best to help you make the diagnosis?

A. AP and lateral x-rays
B. MRI
C. Physical exam only
D. Ortho referral
E. Sed rate and CBC

276.

All of the following would cause concern <u>except</u>:

A. Increased genu valgum in a 3-year-old
B. Persistence of genu valgum in an 8-year-old
C. Genu valgum in a 15-month-old
D. Asymmetric valgus
E. Tibiofemoral angle more than 15 degrees valgus

277.

A mother brings her 3-year-old daughter, Sarah, to see you because she hasn't used her left arm for the last couple of hours. They were at the park when Sarah fell while holding her mother's hand.

On physical examination, she is holding her left arm close to her body with the hand in a pronated position in front of her body and refuses to use it. The wrist and shoulder seem to be normal, but she does experience pain when you try to move the elbow. No tenderness to palpation of her wrist, arm, or elbow.

Which of the following would you do next?

A. Order x-rays before doing anything.
B. Supinate the forearm and then flex the elbow.
C. Consult an orthopedic surgeon immediately.
D. Splint the arm for 5–7 days to immobilize it.
E. Just have mother give ibuprofen and ice the arm for the next several days.

GASTROENTEROLOGY

278.

Niacin (B₃) deficiency does <u>not</u> result in which of the following?

A. Diarrhea
B. Dementia
C. Dermatitis
D. Dyskinesia

279.

Refeeding syndrome is characterized by which of the following?

A. Decreased phosphate
B. Increased potassium
C. Decreased calcium
D. Increased magnesium

280.

Which of the following is currently one of the best screening tests for celiac disease?

A. Anti-gliadin IgG
B. Anti-tissue transglutaminase IgA
C. Anti-gliadin IgA
D. Anti-reticulin IgA

281.

Omphalocele is associated with which of the following?

A. Congenital herniation to the right of the umbilicus
B. Thickened and shortened intestines
C. Other congenital anomalies
D. Exposed small intestines

282.

Which of the following gastrointestinal diseases is <u>not</u> more common in children with Down syndrome?

A. Meckel diverticulum
B. Imperforate anus
C. Duodenal atresia
D. Celiac disease

283.

In a suspected appendicitis, which of the following is the most appropriate therapy?

A. Intravenous fluids
B. Emergency surgery
C. Intravenous antibiotics
D. Repeated examinations

284.

In a child with rectal prolapse, which diagnostic test should be considered?

A. Serum electrolytes
B. Colonoscopy
C. Sweat chloride
D. Rectal suction biopsy

285.

To prevent neural tube defects, pregnant women should have adequate intake of which of the following?

A. Vitamin C
B. Vitamin D
C. Riboflavin
D. Vitamin B_{12}

286.

Why should a choledochal cyst be resected?

A. It is a cancer risk.
B. It is a source of cholestasis.
C. It is a source of infection.
D. It is a source of chronic inflammation.

287.

A school-aged child is found on laboratory testing to have a mildly elevated unconjugated bilirubin. The parents reveal that when ill the child will become mildly jaundiced. The jaundice resolves when the illness is over.

This child most likely has which of the following?

A. Crigler-Najjar syndrome Type 2
B. Gilbert syndrome
C. Hepatitis C
D. Autoimmune hepatitis

288.

On the 5th day of hospitalization for treatment of severe anorexia nervosa associated with a 21% weight loss over an 11-month period of time, a 16-year-old girl complains of difficulty breathing. Although her physician initially thought that she was simply attempting to manipulate the staff to remove her feeding tube, her physical exam reveals a new gallop rhythm associated with bibasilar rales and a respiratory rate of 44 breaths/minute.

Which of the following laboratory findings is the most likely cause of this patient's cardiopulmonary symptoms and findings?

   A. Hypermagnesemia
   B. Hyponatremia
   C. Hyperkalemia
   D. Hypophosphatemia
   E. Hypercalcemia

289.

A 3-year-old Caucasian female is referred for evaluation of failure to thrive. Her parents describe her as "sickly." She has been hospitalized twice for pneumonia. Several months ago she underwent surgery for placement of tympanostomy tubes due to recurrent otitis media. Her parents also describe frequent episodes of foul smelling loose stools. On physical examination, height and weight are at the 5th percentile. Laboratory results include an absolute neutrophil count of 1,100, platelet count of 50,000, and a normal sweat chloride test that, when repeated a second time, was again normal.

Of the following findings, which is most likely to be identified upon further evaluation of this patient?

   A. Bilateral absence of the thumbs
   B. Flattening of the external ears associated with preauricular pitting
   C. Scoliosis associated with sphenoid dysplasia
   D. Mediastinal lymphadenopathy on chest x-ray
   E. Bilateral irregularities of the proximal and distal femoral metaphyses

290.

An 8-year-old Caucasian female presents for a scheduled health maintenance examination. Her growth chart reveals that her weight has decreased over 5 pounds since her last visit a year earlier. Her mother reports that 2 family members have recently been diagnosed with celiac disease.

If the anti-tissue transglutaminase antibody level is normal, which of the following laboratory tests should you order next when evaluating a patient for celiac disease?

   A. Serum total IgA levels
   B. Serum amylase and lipase levels
   C. Pyridoxine (vitamin B₆) levels
   D. Riboflavin (vitamin B₂) levels
   E. Total IgG levels

291.

The parents of a 14-month-old child present to the emergency room with the concern that their son has not had a wet diaper in more than 12 hours. They describe him as having frequent episodes of loose stools, several of which appeared to have contained blood. He is irritable and pale on physical examination. Laboratory findings include elevated levels of blood urea nitrogen (BUN) and creatinine. He is hospitalized for dehydration and possible sepsis. A stool culture is subsequently positive for *Escherichia coli* O157:H7.

Which of the following laboratory findings is likely to be identified during additional evaluation of this patient?

    A. Helmet and burr cells on a peripheral smear
    B. Thrombocytosis
    C. Decrease in serum levels of C3 and CH50
    D. Elevated antistreptolysin O (ASO) titers
    E. Elevated antideoxyribonuclease B titer (Anti-DNAse B)

292.

A 17-year-old female presents to the emergency room with a 4-hour history of severe abdominal pain associated with nausea and vomiting and subjective fever. Her parents describe her as depressed over a recent breakup with her boyfriend. The pain is described as consistent and "deep inside," sometimes radiating to the back and flanks. There is no history of trauma. On physical examination her temperature is 101.4° F. Heart rate is 120, respiratory rate is 28, and blood pressure is 150/98. Her abdomen is diffusely tender, with guarding, especially when palpating the upper quadrants. A periumbilical bluish discoloration is also noted.

Which of the following laboratory findings is likely to be identified during further evaluation of this patient?

    A. Elevated serum amylase and lipase levels
    B. Numerous bacteria and white blood cells on microscopic examination of the urine
    C. Burr and helmet cells on a peripheral smear
    D. Renal calculi on abdominal CT scan
    E. Ruptured ovarian cyst on abdominal ultrasound

293.

The parents of a 3-week-old girl describe recurrent episodes during which time their daughter "gets stiff and arches her back." Oftentimes she will "scream" during such episodes and "look like she is staring into space." Her parents report that she usually "gets stiff" about 20 minutes after breastfeeding and will cry intermittently for an hour or so thereafter. She routinely feeds for 10 minutes at each breast. Her birth history is benign. She takes no medications and has gained 15 ounces since birth.

Which of the following is the most likely cause of this patient's symptoms?

    A. Cyanotic breath holding spells
    B. Pallid breath holding spells
    C. Gastroesophageal reflux
    D. Anomalous coronary artery
    E. Infantile spasms

294.

The parents of a 10-month-old boy present with the concern that their son "has yellow jaundice." They report that he is otherwise well with the exception that his stools are a little more frequent. On physical exam his skin has a yellowish hue, most prominent on the palms, soles, cheeks, and tip of his nose. His conjunctivas are clear.

Which of the following is likely to provide the explanation for this patient's clinical findings?

A. Abdominal ultrasound
B. Hepatitis panel
C. Liver biopsy
D. Dietary history
E. Sending stool for fat and reducing substances

295.

A 16-year-old male is admitted to a psychiatric hospital because of severe depression. He has not responded to outpatient intervention, which included counseling and treatment with an antidepressant. His physical examination is positive for a depressed affect and a parkinsonian-like tremor. During routine laboratory evaluation he is found to have unexpected elevations in serum aminotransferases and bilirubin concentrations.

Which of the following is most likely to be abnormal during additional evaluation of this patient?

A. A slit-lamp examination
B. A bone marrow biopsy
C. A renal ultrasound
D. A 24-hour urine for protein
E. The opening pressure as measured during lumbar puncture

296.

A 6-year-old girl presents with a 3-day history of low-grade fever, abdominal cramping, and diarrhea. Several of her classmates have similar symptoms. She is otherwise well and takes no daily medications. On physical examination she has a temperature of 101.1° F and her blood pressure is 100/65 mmHg. Her mucus membranes are moist. Capillary refill is < 3 seconds. Her abdomen is moderately tender throughout. Bowel sounds are hyperactive. There is no evidence of rebound tenderness. A stool culture is obtained, which grows *Salmonella typhimurium*.

Which of the following is the most appropriate next step in the treatment of this patient?

A. Oral amoxicillin
B. Intramuscular ceftriaxone
C. Oral trimethoprim-sulfamethoxazole
D. Symptomatic treatment only
E. Oral erythromycin

297.

A 20-month-old boy presents to the emergency room after several episodes of bloody diarrhea. His parents deny associated symptoms of fever, appetite change, or decrease in activity. Several months prior to presentation he had several bloody stools, which were thought to be associated with a "bad stomach virus" and cleared spontaneously. On physical examination he is afebrile, alert, playful, and interactive. His abdominal exam is positive only for increased bowel sounds. A stool sample is positive for blood.

Which of the following is the most likely cause of this patient's clinical signs and symptoms?

    A. Ectopic gastric tissue
    B. Invagination of a part of the intestine into itself
    C. An area(s) of erosion within the gastric mucosa
    D. *Helicobacter pylori* located within the stomach and duodenum
    E. Increased production of gastrin from a duodenal gastrinoma

298.

The parents of a 4-month-old girl present to the emergency room after their daughter had a "2-minute period of stiffening while staring with her head to the right and arching her back." They also express concern that their daughter appeared to have briefly "stopped breathing." They deny associated cyanosis. She is described as "a generally fussy baby" but has no known medical problems. They have, however, noticed that she will sometimes "keep her head turned to one side or the other and cry." On physical examination she is in the 55th percentile for height, weight and head circumference. She is afebrile and has no abnormal findings on exam.

Which of the following is the most likely cause of intermittent torticollis in this patient?

    A. Gastroesophageal reflux
    B. Atlantoaxial instability
    C. Arnold-Chiari malformation
    D. Clavicular fracture
    E. Posterior fossa tumor

299.

A hospitalized 6-year-old boy complains of right upper quadrant pain. An abdominal ultrasound shows prominent noncalculous distention of the gallbladder. Findings on physical examination include a rash.

Which of the following best describes the rash most commonly associated with this patient's findings on abdominal ultrasound?

    A. A widespread morbilliform rash that is particularly prominent in the perineum and intertriginous areas
    B. A rash consisting of petechial and purpuric coalescent lesions involving the buttocks and lower extremities
    C. An erythematous rash in a malar distribution that spares the nasolabial folds
    D. Numerous small brownish papules and plaques that react to stroking with a wheel and flare-type reaction
    E. A maculopapular rash associated with numerous petechiae involving the wrists, palms, ankles and soles and, to a lesser extent, the trunk

300.

A 4-week-old previously healthy Caucasian male presents to your clinic with a 4-day history of vomiting that has gotten progressively worse. His mother reports the vomitus just looks like milk—there is no yellow or green in it. At first the vomiting occurred only every once in a while, but now it seems to be after almost every feeding and is more forceful.

REVIEW OF SYSTEMS: There has been no fever or diarrhea, and actually, the number of stools has decreased. No cold symptoms.

PAST MEDICAL HISTORY: Healthy term infant born to G1 mother. No complications.

ALLERGIES: NKDA

FAMILY HISTORY: Grandmother with Crohn disease, otherwise negative

PHYSICAL EXAMINATION:
T 99° F, HR 155, BP 90/65
General: Alert but fussy.

HEENT: Anterior fontanel flat; TMs and nose clear; OP clear except sticky mucous membranes
Heart: Regular, no murmurs
Lungs: Clear
Abd: + bowel sounds, soft with small mass in midepigastric area
Ext: Pulses 2+

After a definitive diagnosis is made with appropriate tests and labs, which of the following would you select as your next step?

A. Instruct mother that this is a viral illness and to give Pedialyte® for the next 24 hours at home.
B. Give IVF but omit KCl since most likely this child has a high potassium level and is acidotic.
C. Send him to surgery immediately.
D. Give IVF with 20–40 mEq/L KCl to correct electrolyte/acid-base imbalance.
E. Instruct mother that she is overfeeding this infant and should decrease the amount/feeding.

301.

A 17-year-old Caucasian female presents to your office with a 2-month history of bloody stools. Occasionally they are loose but usually are large, bulky stools. She has had crampy abdominal pain on and off for 6 months. No fever or vomiting. She does seem to tire easily.

PAST MEDICAL HISTORY: She has been very healthy except has had a lot of oral aphthous ulcers.

IMMUNIZATIONS: UTD

FAMILY HISTORY: Paternal grandmother had several autoimmune diseases, but patient unsure which ones—did involve the liver.

SOCIAL HISTORY: Has city water. No recent travel. Family owns cattle. No new pets.

On physical examination, she is at the 75th percentile for both weight and height, although she has lost 5 pounds in the last couple of months. Vital signs are stable. Everything looks normal except she has mild discomfort to palpation of abdomen. Rectal reveals heme + stool. No anal fissures visualized.

You treat her for constipation for 1 month without relief of symptoms. You order lab work that shows normal WBC count and sedimentation rate. Hematocrit is 30%. Stool cultures, and ova and parasites, are negative. You then send her to the gastroenterologist for colonoscopy, which shows multiple linear ulcers and fistulas. Rectum appears normal. There are multiple patchy areas of erythema with normal mucosa in between.

Which of the following is the most likely diagnosis?

   A. Crohn disease
   B. Ulcerative colitis
   C. Infectious colitis
   D. Enteric parasites
   E. Systemic lupus erythematosus

302.

A 5-year-old girl presents with a history of diarrhea for 2 days. She has had fever with the diarrhea to 102° F. Her stools this morning had frank blood in them, which prompted her parents to bring her in. She has a new pet puppy, which she received about a month ago. The puppy has not been ill.

Cultures of the stool show motile, comma-shaped Gram-negative bacilli.

Which of the following is the most likely organism?

   A. *Campylobacter jejuni*
   B. *Shigella sonnei*
   C. *Salmonella* species
   D. Ameba
   E. *Bartonella henselae*

303.

You are seeing a 9-month-old Caucasian male for follow-up of diarrhea. It started at 4 months of age after his mother started him on solids. He has been on the same formula since birth and had no problems the first 4 months. For the past 5 months, he has had vomiting off and on, decreased appetite, irritability, and periodic abdominal distention.

On physical examination, he has dropped to the 10th percentile from the 50th percentile at 4 months. Length remains at the 25th percentile. There is mild muscle wasting, but the rest of the exam is normal.

You've already ordered lab tests on a previous visit, including stool for culture, and ova and parasites, both of which are negative. His hematocrit is 30% and albumin is slightly low.

Which of the following is the next lab you would order?

A. Growth hormone
B. Thyroid function tests
C. Zinc level
D. Anti-transglutaminase IgA antibodies
E. CPK and aldolase

304.

A 16-year-old Caucasian male with a history of acne is brought in by his mother because of the acute onset of difficulty swallowing this morning. He has had continued difficulty since breakfast. He notes nothing unusual before this and had a good night's sleep. He says school is going very well, and he really enjoys being in the band. He did not notice a problem until he tried to eat his breakfast, which consisted of a chocolate pop tart and tortilla chips.

PAST MEDICAL HISTORY: Acne for about 2 years treated with topical agents initially and now on doxycycline 100 mg PO bid for the past 3 months. He has been adherent to his medication regimen and took the medication this morning.

REVIEW OF SYSTEMS: No fever, chills, night sweats
                         Has difficulty swallowing—only solids, not liquids
                         No nausea or vomiting
                         No diarrhea
                         No skin changes

PHYSICAL EXAMINATION:
Well-developed, obese WM in no apparent distress
BP 130/70, P 90, RR 16, Temp 98.5° F, Height 5'10", Weight 250 lbs

HEENT:	PERRLA, EOMI
	No oral thrush
	No abnormalities seen
Neck:	Supple, non-tender examination
Heart:	RRR with 2/6 systolic flow murmur (not new, heard in the past)
Lungs:	CTA
Abdomen:	Bowel sounds heard in all quadrants; no hepatosplenomegaly
Extremities:	No cyanosis, clubbing, or edema
Skin:	Acne is very mild compared to 3 months ago; no back lesions at present

Which of the following is the most likely etiology of his swallowing complaint?

A. Pill-induced esophagitis
B. Gastroesophageal reflux
C. Scleroderma
D. Cocaine abuse
E. Bulimia

305.

A 1-month-old presents with newly found cholestatic jaundice. Her stools are bile stained.

Which of the following is the next procedure that should be performed?

- A. Ultrasound
- B. Hepatic scintigraphy
- C. Chromosomal analysis
- D. Hepatitis panel
- E. Percutaneous liver biopsy

306.

A 15-year-old female presents with a history of recurrent diarrhea. Recently she has become concerned because the diarrhea has occurred while she is sleeping. Additionally, she notes that she has had abdominal pain on occasion. The pain is relieved by defecation. Usually the pain is located in the right lower quadrant. She describes it as a chronic nagging type pain ("colicky"). On further questioning, she relates that she has had about a 10 lb. weight loss over the past 5 months. Her mother has noted that she sweats "a lot" during the night and occasionally she has had to change her bedclothes because of it. Also, she reports that on occasion she is "feverish" but has not taken her temperature. She has not traveled anywhere outside of Colorado where she lives, although, she did go camping during the past summer at Pike's Peak. Her last camping trip was 3 months ago. They boiled water while camping and did not go swimming. No one else has been ill.

PAST MEDICAL HISTORY: History of frequent episodes of diarrhea intermittently over the past 5 years

ALLERGIES: None

FAMILY HISTORY: Mother with episodes of diarrhea on occasion
Father with coronary artery disease, hypertension
Sister healthy, no problems
Brother healthy, no problems

SOCIAL HISTORY: Attends 10th grade at local high school
Lives with mother, father, 2 siblings, and 2 dogs in the city limits
Dogs are healthy, no problems
Never has smoked
Doesn't drink

REVIEW OF SYSTEMS: Most reviewed above
No blood noted in stool
Stools of normal caliber when she is not having diarrhea

PHYSICAL EXAMINATION:
Well appearing adolescent in no distress
BP 110/65, P 68, RR 16, Temp 99.2° F

HEENT: PERRLA, EOMI
Throat normal
Normal dentition

Neck:	Supple, no thyromegaly
Heart:	RRR without murmurs, rubs, or gallops
Lungs:	CTA
Abdomen:	Bowel sounds hyperactive, present in all 4 quadrants equally
	Mild epigastric discomfort with deep palpation; no rebound
	No Hepatosplenomegaly
Extremities:	No cyanosis, clubbing, or edema
GU:	Normal female genitalia
	Heme positive rectal exam

LABORATORY:

CBC: WBC 12,500 with 60% polys, 20% lymphocytes, 15% monocytes
Hemoglobin 10.5 g/dL
Platelets: 450,000

Stool Studies: Marked number of fecal leukocytes seen on direct smear; Negative for enteric pathogens, ova and parasites, *Giardia* specific antigen, and *Clostridium difficile* toxin.

Electrolytes:	Normal
Liver transaminases:	Normal for age
ESR:	50

Based on your history and physical examination, which of the following studies is most likely to confirm your diagnosis?

A. MRI of the abdomen and pelvis
B. Endoscopic laparotomy
C. Repeat ova and parasite studies x 3
D. Rectal biopsy
E. Air contrast barium enema and enteroclysis

307.

Which of the following is true with regard to "breast-milk" jaundice?

A. Jaundice never persists longer than 1 month.
B. Kernicterus can occur at a rate of 10%.
C. Infants with breast-milk jaundice are usually less vigorous.
D. The serum bilirubin reaches maximum concentrations of 15 to 25 mg/dL during the 2nd or 3rd week.
E. The jaundice is due to conjugated and unconjugated bilirubin.

308.

Which of the following is true with regard to "physiologic jaundice" of the newborn?

A. Serum bilirubin reaches maximum values near 6 mg/dL between the 1st and 2nd week in full-term infants.
B. Physiologic jaundice can cause damage in healthy full-term neonates approximately 10% of the time.
C. Serum bilirubin reaches maximum values near 6 mg/dL between the 2nd and 4th day in full-term infants.
D. The excess bilirubin is due to increased bilirubin in breast milk.
E. Pigment concentrations decline gradually and reach normal values in 5–7 days in term infants.

309.

A 16-year-old hip-hop singer has been ill with diarrhea for the past 2 weeks. She says that she noted this while she was performing in Mexico. You are the physician for the cruise line that she is performing for now. You really like her song, "OOPS, I'm going again." But we digress from the topic at hand ….

Anyway, she tells you that she has had some low-grade temperatures since returning from Mexico. She did not eat any fresh vegetables, unless you call French fries a fresh vegetable. She likes to eat beef jerky and prefers the "extra salty" version. She drank only bottled water and a soft drink for which she is a national spokesperson. She did drink these drinks poured over ice; however, she thought that the "frozen stuff would kill the cooties."

She has not noted any blood in her stool. She has lost about 2 pounds in the last week.

PAST MEDICAL HISTORY:	Syphilis at the age of 15
	Depression since age 14, on no medications at the moment
SOCIAL HISTORY:	Sexually active with multiple partners
	Smokes 1 pack/day for the past 3 years
	Denies illicit drug use
	Denies use of alcohol
FAMILY HISTORY:	Mother with alcoholism; they are estranged at the moment
	Father left when she was 2 years of age
	Sister healthy 20-year-old nun
REVIEW OF SYSTEMS:	Diarrhea is intermittent and she has crampy abdominal pain on occasion
	No rash
	No burning on urination
	No chills
	Diminished appetite

PHYSICAL EXAMINATION:
General: Pink hair with numerous piercings
Temp 100.0° F, BP 110/70, P 95, RR 16

HEENT:	PERRLA, EOMI
	Throat clear
Heart:	RRR with no murmurs, rubs, or gallops;
Lungs:	CTA
Abdomen:	Hyperactive bowel sounds, non-tender examination; no hepatosplenomegaly
GU:	Normal female genitalia, no tenderness on bi-manual palpation; no discharge noted
Extremities:	No cyanosis, clubbing, or edema
Rectal:	Heme positive (slight)

LABORATORY:

Check for stool leukocytes:	Positive
Giardia specific antigen:	Negative
Stool culture:	*Salmonella enteritidis* Beta lactamase producing

Based on this information, which of the following is the best treatment?

A. No antibiotic therapy
B. Ciprofloxacin 500 mg bid for 10 days
C. Erythromycin 500 mg bid for 5 days
D. Tetracycline 500 mg qid for 10 days
E. Amoxicillin 500 mg tid for 10 days

310.

A 16-year-old lifeguard at the local water park in your area presents for his final hepatitis B vaccine and routine examination. Recently there has been an outbreak of diarrhea at the water park confirmed as *E. coli* O157:H7. He is concerned about the diarrhea at the park and asks about what he can do to limit his exposure. You explain that the outbreak has been linked to hamburgers at the park that were undercooked. He is concerned because he eats hamburgers twice daily. You explain that it is unlikely that he will become ill but to call you at the first sign of diarrhea.

The next morning you receive a call from him saying that he has diarrhea. It is bloody in character. You tell him to come in right away.

He arrives and is ill-appearing. He says the diarrhea started early this morning and he has gone about 5 times since. He noted large amounts of blood in the initial stool, but it has since tapered off to a few streaks. He says he is lightheaded and is dizzy.

PAST MEDICAL HISTORY: Healthy

SOCIAL HISTORY: As above
                         Doesn't smoke
                         Doesn't drink alcohol
                         Not sexually active

FAMILY HISTORY: Non-contributory

REVIEW OF SYSTEMS: Fever, chills noted early this morning
                         Weight loss of approximately 5 pounds since yesterday, he thinks
                         Dizzy when standing
                         No vomiting

PHYSICAL EXAMINATION:
Lying down: BP 120/80, P 80
Sitting up: BP 100/65, P 110
T 99.5° F, RR 18

HEENT: PERRLA, EOMI,
              Tympanic membranes clear
              Throat clear; mucous membranes dry
Neck: Supple, no bruits
Heart: RRR without murmurs, rubs, or gallops
Lungs: CTA
Abdomen: Benign, no tenderness, no hepatosplenomegaly
Extremities: No cyanosis, clubbing, or edema

Neurological: Reflexes equal and symmetrical throughout, no sensory or motor deficits noted
Rectal: Heme-positive stool

LABORATORY: All pending

Assuming that this is invasive diarrhea with *E. coli* O157:H7, and after starting supportive fluid therapy, which of the following antibiotics is the best choice for treatment of his infection?

A. Penicillin 3 million units IV q 4 hours
B. Ceftriaxone 1 gm IV q day
C. Await sensitivities before starting therapy
D. Ciprofloxacin 400 mg IV bid
E. None of the choices are correct

311.

You have been asked to consult in the hospital on a 15-year-old Caucasian male with new onset of a debilitating neurological syndrome. He has been healthy until about a month ago, when he had gastroenteritis. He says the gastroenteritis lasted about a week and then resolved without any specific therapy. Most of the disease was a diarrheal illness. He has a puppy that also had diarrhea just before he became ill. The patient's diarrhea was bloody in character, and he had crampy abdominal pain. His diarrhea lasted about 5 days. The dog's disease also lasted about that long.

He noted painless onset of mild weakness in the lower extremities, often accompanied by tingling paresthesias in his toes and fingers. He first became aware of this with difficulty walking up stairs. Over a period of days, the weakness progressed rapidly and ascended from the lower extremities to the upper extremities and finally to the face.

PAST MEDICAL HISTORY: Noncontributory

SOCIAL HISTORY:
Attends local high school
Smokes 3 cigarettes a day
Drinks rarely on weekends; about a 6-pack of beer when he does
No travel history

FAMILY HISTORY: Non-contributory

REVIEW OF SYSTEM:
No fevers, no chills
No weight loss
No recent diarrhea (after original episode resolved)
No vomiting
No rashes
No headache
No vision changes

PHYSICAL EXAMINATION:
BP 110/70, P100, RR 18, Temp 98.5° F

HEENT:
PERRLA, EOMI,
Tympanic membranes clear
Throat clear

Neck:	Supple, no bruits
Heart:	RRR without murmurs, rubs, or gallops
Lungs:	CTA
Abdomen:	Benign, no tenderness, no hepatosplenomegaly
Extremities:	No cyanosis, clubbing, or edema
Neurological:	Deep tendon reflexes are not present
	He has lost proprioceptive perception in his arms and legs
	He has symmetrical motor weakness of both proximal and distal muscles of all the extremities
	He has bilateral VII nerve palsies
	Currently swallowing and breathing are intact

Which of the following is the likely antecedent to this constellation of findings?

A. *Campylobacter jejuni*
B. *Shigella dysenteriae*
C. *Salmonella enteritidis*
D. *E. coli* O157:H7
E. Rotavirus infection

312.

A 16-year-old Caucasian girl presents with a history of chronic diarrhea for over a year. She has complained of diarrhea on many visits to your office. Listed below is the laboratory work that has been done to date, including a few tests done today. The diarrhea is intermittent in character, lasts 3–5 days, and then her stools gradually return to normal. She has not noticed any blood in the stool. She has no nausea or vomiting. She has no other health problems. Her boyfriend and her 1-year-old child, who live with her, have had no problems with diarrhea. She has not had significant weight loss. The stools are not foul smelling and are usually fairly watery in character.

PAST MEDICAL HISTORY:	History of depression at age 15 requiring hospitalization; since then doing well on Prozac 20 mg q day
SOCIAL HISTORY:	Beauty college student Smokes 1/2 pack/day for 3 years Alcohol—doesn't drink
FAMILY HISTORY:	Mother healthy, no health problems Father healthy, no health problems Sister, anorexia Brother, bulimia
REVIEW OF SYSTEMS:	No fever, chills No sore throats No increased nervousness No chest discomfort No wheezing No stomach pain No rashes No travel

PHYSICAL EXAMINATION:
Well-appearing Caucasian female, with excessive amounts of makeup
BP 120/60, P 64, RR18, Temp 98.3° F

HEENT:	PERRLA, EOMI, sclera non-icteric
Neck:	Supple; no masses
Heart:	RRR without murmurs, rubs, or gallops
Lungs:	Clear to auscultation
Abdomen:	Mild epigastric tenderness to deep palpation
Extremities:	No cyanosis, clubbing, or edema
GU:	Heme-negative stool; scant amount of stool in vault

LABORATORY:

CBC x 2:	Normal
Electrolytes x 3:	Normal
Liver transaminases x 2:	Normal
Stool ova and parasites and fecal leukocytes x 3:	Negative
C. difficile toxin:	Negative
Chem 20:	Normal
TSH:	Normal
T4:	Normal
Gastrin level:	Normal
Giardia specific antigen:	Negative
Sigmoidoscopy:	Negative
Sodium hydroxide added to stool:	Turns red

Based on your findings, which of the following do the history, physical and laboratory findings suggest?

A. Bisacodyl abuse
B. Phenolphthalein abuse
C. Irritable bowel syndrome (IBS)
D. Carcinoid
E. Need to proceed with colonoscopy

313.

Your patient is a 17-year-old Irish-American with history of celiac sprue. He has been compliant with his diet. He was not diagnosed until several years ago. This resulted in growth retardation as a child. He currently plays a leprechaun in a revival of "Finian's Rainbow." He occasionally suffers from dermatitis herpetiformis. He comes in today for routine checkup and complains of increasing fatigue over the past 3 months. He has a pale pallor to his skin, and he looks "run down" to you.

PAST MEDICAL HISTORY:	As above
MEDICATIONS:	None
SOCIAL HISTORY:	Works in theater as a leprechaun
	Has never smoked
	Doesn't drink alcohol
FAMILY HISTORY:	Sister has celiac sprue also; found to have HLA-B8
	Mother and father healthy

REVIEW OF SYSTEMS: Severe fatigue
Dyspnea on exertion with walking 1 block
No chest pain
No swelling in his legs
No constipation

PHYSICAL EXAMINATION:
BP 120/60, P 100, RR18, Temp 99.0° F

HEENT:	PERRLA, EOMI, sclera non-icteric, very pale conjunctiva
Neck:	Supple; no bruits; no masses
Heart:	RRR with new II/VI systolic flow murmur
Lungs:	Clear to auscultation
Abdomen:	Mild epigastric tenderness to deep palpation
Extremities:	No cyanosis, clubbing, or edema
GU:	Heme-negative stool

LABORATORY:
    CBC: WBC 8,500 with 60% polys, 30% lymphs
Hemoglobin 8.5 mg/dL (this low value is **new**)
Rest of CBC pending ... the machine just broke

Which of the following is the most likely reason for his fatigue?

A. Iron deficiency anemia
B. B$_{12}$ deficiency anemia
C. Toxicity from wearing green leprechaun paint
D. Celiac sprue exacerbation
E. Primary intestinal lymphoma

314.

A 16-year-old Caucasian female with history of abdominal complaints off and on "for years" presents with acute onset of severe pain in her left abdomen. She has fever to 101° F at home and appears ill. She has had some associated diarrhea with the pain.

PAST MEDICAL HISTORY: History of GI disease. See figure below from colonoscopy from last year

SOCIAL HISTORY: Junior in high school. Lives at home with her parents

REVIEW OF SYSTEMS: No headache
No sore throat
No runny nose; congestion
Occasional dry cough
No tachycardia
No chest pain
No constipation
Diarrhea frequently, usually with emotional upset
No burning on urination

PHYSICAL EXAMINATION:
BP 130/88, P 100, RR 18, Temp 101.5° F
Ill appearing in mild distress

HEENT:	PERRLA, EOMI
	TM's clear
	Throat clear
Neck:	Supple; no masses
Heart:	RRR without murmurs, rubs, or gallops
Lungs:	Clear to auscultation
Abdomen:	Hyperactive bowel sounds; tender and palpable mass in left lower quadrant; rebound tenderness noted and involuntary abdominal rigidity noted
Rectal:	Heme-positive
Extremities:	No rashes, cyanosis, or edema

LABORATORY: Pending

Which of the following should be done at this point?

A. Emergent colonoscopy
B. Emergent barium enema
C. Bowel rest only is adequate at this point
D. Abdominal CT scan
E. Bleeding scan

315.

A 10-year-old boy with a long history of asthma is admitted to the Intensive Care Unit with severe respiratory failure. He requires intubation, ventilatory support, bronchodilators, and IV corticosteroids. He has no other medical problems. After 3 days of therapy, the critical care physicians are able to extubate the patient. However, once there is initiation of oral feedings, the patient complains of severe pain while swallowing. Upper endoscopy is performed and reveals multiple shallow small ulcers in the distal esophagus. Biopsies are pending at this time.

Which of the following is the <u>least</u> likely diagnosis?

A. Reflux esophagitis
B. Herpes esophagitis
C. *Candida* esophagitis
D. Pill-induced esophagitis
E. Mechanical injury related to nasogastric tube

316.

A 15-year-old patient with ulcerative colitis, who has been in clinical remission for the past year on mesalamine, develops diarrhea and abdominal pain. She denies rectal bleeding. This is similar to past flares of the colitis except for the lack of bleeding.

PAST MEDICAL HISTORY: Ulcerative colitis on mesalamine 2.4 gm per day

REVIEW OF SYSTEMS: Recent abscessed tooth that required 5 days of clindamycin. Complains of occasional joint pain.

PHYSICAL EXAMINATION:
T 99° F, no apparent distress.
Abdomen is soft and nontender, although slightly distended.

LAB TESTS: Hgb 12.0, WBC 15,500

Which of the following would you recommend?

    A. Admit to the hospital for IV corticosteroids and careful monitoring for possible toxic megacolon.
    B. Check for fecal leukocytes and if positive, treat with metronidazole.
    C. Perform an unprepped flexible sigmoidoscopy to assess for pseudomembranes.
    D. Check the stool for *Clostridium difficile* toxin before initiating therapy.
    E. Send a stool culture for *Clostridium difficile.*

317.

4 adults and 2 children present to the Emergency Room, all within 30 minutes of each other, exhibiting similar symptoms. They all describe the sudden onset of nausea and severe vomiting. Shortly thereafter, all of them developed profuse diarrhea, and now all complain of severe weakness. All 6 people had been together that afternoon, because they (or their parents) all work for a company in Colorado Springs that provides study material for doctors taking Board exams. The company was celebrating the summer with a picnic. There was a variety of different foods that were brought by different people, including "Marla's famous" deviled eggs, ham sandwiches, sashimi, barbecued chicken, hamburgers on the grill, as well as raspberries and melon balls. None of the people involved remember eating any other items. All had been swimming in a creek and 2 admit to possibly ingesting some of the creek water. The nausea started almost exactly 4 hours after the picnic.

On presentation to the Emergency Room, the person complaining of the most profound weakness has a blood pressure of 80/40 with a heart rate of 140 and decreased skin turgor. Temperature is 97° F. Abdomen is soft and nontender. IV fluids have been started.

Which of the following is <u>true</u>?

    A. This is probable *Salmonella* related to undercooking of poultry.
    B. This is likely giardiasis from drinking the creek water in Colorado, which is commonly infested with *Giardia.*
    C. This is likely *E. coli* O157:H7 related to the undercooked hamburger.
    D. This is likely a *Staphylococcus aureus* food poisoning.
    E. This is likely not due to Marla's deviled eggs or any other food at the picnic.

318.

Which of the following is true with regard to organic and functional abdominal pain in children?

A. Pain farther from the umbilicus is more likely organic.
B. Crampy abdominal pain is more likely organic.
C. Night awakening is not common with functional abdominal pain.
D. Duration of pain is helpful in discerning between the two.
E. Associated diarrhea is common in functional pain.

319.

A 9-month-old Caucasian male is awakened from a sound sleep with severe crampy abdominal pain and flexion of his knees and hips. The pain abates spontaneously and he appears normal. A few minutes later, though, the pain recurs. He starts to vomit, and he has a normal bowel movement. However, his parents then note that he has a dark red, bloody, "cranberry-like" material pass in his diaper. A small abdominal mass is palpated in the right upper and middle quadrants.

A contrast enema is scheduled.

Which of the following is a contraindication to performing the therapeutic enema?

A. Fever
B. Vomiting
C. Diarrhea
D. Eating within the previous hour
E. Peritoneal inflammation

320.

Which of the following is <u>not</u> true about Meckel diverticulum?

A. Occurs in 2% of the population.
B. It is usually within 2 cm of the ileocecal valve.
C. Is the most common GI anomaly.
D. Painless rectal bleeding most often occurs in the 2-year-old age group.
E. The diagnostic sensitivity of radionucleotide scanning can be improved with prior administration of an H_2-blocker.

321.

You are seeing a first-born male for his 2-month immunizations and well-child checkup. It was noted in the nursery that he had delay in passage of meconium. He is growing well, and his mother notes that he has bowel movements, but that they are intermittent and he may go several days without one. His examination shows a distended abdomen with a palpable stool mass. His anal canal and rectum are empty with no palpable fecal material. Hirschsprung disease is high on your differential (darn, weren't you hoping that was the answer to the question?).

Which of the following is seen in Hirschsprung disease?

A. On barium enema, the aganglionic segment is the proximal narrowed segment and the normal ganglionic segment is dilated distally.
B. On barium enema, the aganglionic segment is the distal narrowed segment and the normal ganglionic segment is dilated proximally.
C. On barium enema, the aganglionic segment is the proximal dilated segment and the ganglionic segment is the distal narrowed segment.
D. On barium enema, the aganglionic segment is the distal dilated segment and the ganglionic segment is narrowed proximally.
E. A rectal biopsy is always indicated.

322.

A 15-year-old Caucasian male with negative past medical history presents with the chief complaint of "turning yellow." He noticed that he was becoming yellow in his eyes yesterday. Today he said that his skin is also yellow. He has no nausea, vomiting, or other complaints.

PAST MEDICAL HISTORY: Negative

SOCIAL HISTORY:
Works at Taco Ringer as a cook
Lives with his girlfriend of 3 months
Became sexually active and had multiple sexual partners starting one year ago. Has been monogamous for 3 months and 1 day.
Smokes marijuana on weekends
Drinks beer on weekends

REVIEW OF SYSTEMS: Essentially non-contributory

PHYSICAL EXAMINATION:
Only pertinent findings:
Scleral icterus
Liver down about 5 cm and has a span of 17 cm; slightly tender
Spleen tip palpable
No spider angiomas

LABORATORY:
Anti HAV IgM negative
Anti HAV IgG positive
Anti-HBc IgM positive
HBsAg negative
Anti-HBc IgG negative

Which of the following is the correct interpretation of his laboratory data?

A. He has acute hepatitis A and past infection with hepatitis B.
B. He has chronic hepatitis A and acute hepatitis B.
C. He has chronic hepatitis A and chronic hepatitis B.
D. He has acute hepatitis B and past infection with hepatitis A.
E. He has neither hepatitis A nor hepatitis B; he is just antibody positive.

323.

Which of the following is true regarding the treatment of chronic hepatitis C?

A. By attaching a polyethylene glycol moiety to interferon alpha, there is an increased response rate.
B. Interferon alpha given alone 6 million units 3 times a week is more efficacious than when used with ribavirin.
C. Infectious complications related to neutropenia frequently require cessation of antiviral therapy.
D. Patients rarely respond to therapy.
E. HCV genotype I is more responsive to therapy.

324.

An 18-year-old male presents to the office with a chief complaint of fatigue. He has been very distressed and upset since his older brother recently required a liver transplantation for hemochromatosis. He has been told that this disease can be hereditary and that he needs to be "checked out." He is otherwise a healthy young man who has never had any significant medical problems. He takes no medications. On review of systems, he complains of occasional knee pain after tennis.

PHYSICAL EXAMINATION: The skin is normal pigmentation. The sclera is anicteric and there is no sign of jaundice. There is no hepatomegaly or enlargement of the spleen. No ascites felt on exam.
Lab tests included a normal CBC, AST: 28, ALT: 24, alk phos 72.
You consider further testing.

Which of the following statements is true?

A. A serum ferritin of greater than 500 is diagnostic for hereditary hemochromatosis.
B. Transferrin saturation greater than 50% should prompt further evaluation, including *HFE* gene determination.
C. Laboratory tests for iron are notoriously unreliable and therefore not needed. This patient should directly have a liver biopsy looking for hepatic iron concentration.
D. No further testing is necessary with normal laboratories, no hepatomegaly, or abnormal skin color.
E. A serum ferritin of greater than 700 is diagnostic for hereditary hemochromatosis.

325.

Which of the following is the most common cause of acute fulminant liver failure in the United States?

A. Wilson disease
B. Hepatitis B virus
C. Ingestion of amanita species mushrooms
D. Hepatitis C virus
E. Drug hepatotoxicity

GENETICS / METABOLIC DISEASES

326.

A 3-kg infant is born to a mother on lithium for bipolar disease.

Which of the following medical complications is this infant <u>most</u> at risk for?

A. Cardiac malformations
B. Encephalopathy
C. Genitourinary tract malformations
D. Neonatal seizures
E. Neonatal withdrawal syndrome

327.

An 11-year-old male comes in for his sports physical. He is generally healthy but struggles in school and has been in special education classes his whole school career. Both parents are in the normal range for height and have advanced degrees. On physical exam, you notice jittery lenses after he removes his glasses; and he has pectus excavatum. Ht is 170cm (> 97%), Wt is 52kg (90–97%), HC is 50cm (10%), and blood pressure is normal. He has 4 café-au-lait spots, he is prepubertal, and the rest of the exam is unremarkable.

Which of the following is the <u>most</u> likely cause for his tall stature?

A. Familial tall stature
B. Klinefelter syndrome
C. Marfan syndrome
D. Homocystinuria
E. Neurofibromatosis

328.

A girl is brought to your clinic at 20 months because she was slow to start walking and her parents are concerned about her bowed legs. On physical exam she has a prominent forehead—looks like she has craniosynostosis, wide wrists, and is at 3% for height, 10% for weight.

Laboratory shows: Alkaline Phosphatase: 80 (125–300)
Calcium: 12.5 (9.0–11.0)
Vitamin D levels: normal
Phosphate level: normal
PTH: normal
X-rays show rachitic changes with thinning of the bones

Which of the following is the <u>most</u> likely diagnosis?

    A. Familial hypophosphatemic rickets
    B. Osteogenesis imperfecta
    C. Hypophosphatasia
    D. Vitamin D-resistant rickets
    E. Fanconi syndrome

329.

A 3-week-old Hispanic male is brought to clinic because his mother thinks he looks yellow. He has been taking formula well, about 3–4 oz every 3–4 hours. Growth is good, along the 25th percentile. The infant is having the normal number of wet diapers and is stooling, but mother notices that it is greyish compared to her other children. On physical exam you notice moderate icterus; he has a small II/VI holosystolic murmur and a pointed chin with broad forehead. As you get a chest x-ray, you observe butterfly vertebrae at T5. Liver is palpable to 3cm below the costal margin; spleen is not palpable. Lab studies show elevated total and direct bilirubinemia with mild elevations in the liver enzymes. Abdominal ultrasound is unremarkable; no gallbladder was seen.

Which of the following is the most appropriate next management step?

    A. Hemoglobin electrophoresis
    B. Echocardiogram
    C. Sweat test
    D. Urine-reducing substances
    E. Nuclear medicine scan for bile uptake

330.

You are asked by the discharge nurse to see a male infant in the newborn nursery to ascertain recommendations for follow-up. He is a term newborn, doing well and about ready to be discharged home, when the parents start asking about his birthmark on his face. You examine him and find a port-wine stain along the distribution of cranial nerve V on the upper right side of the face.

Which of the following is the <u>most</u> important risk/complication of this finding to discuss with the family?

    A. Hypersplenism
    B. Possible growth and need for steroid injections to decrease swelling over the eyelid
    C. Tethered spinal cord
    D. Glaucoma
    E. Congestive heart failure

331.

An 8-year-old girl has difficulty in academics and a short attention span. Her father states that he had the same problems when he was a child. Physical examination reveals macrocephaly, multiple café-au-lait macules, and axillary freckles. Upon questioning, the father explains that he has similar skin findings.

Which of the following is the most common inheritance pattern for this disorder?

A. Multifactorial
B. X-linked dominant
C. Autosomal dominant
D. Autosomal recessive
E. Mitochondrial

332.

You are called to the newborn nursery to evaluate an infant who has a limb anomaly. The infant is normally grown and vigorous. On physical examination, you note a terminal transverse limb defect at the distal aspect of the right forearm, with absent radius and rudimentary thumb.

Which of the following is the most concerning possible complication?

A. Intracranial hemorrhage
B. Cleft palate
C. Ventricular septal defect
D. Short stature
E. Kidney problems

333.

The pregnant mother of a child in your practice recently learned that her mother had a child who died of "probable metabolic disease" at 2 days of age. She does not know details, and medical records on that child no longer are available. The mother asks if her pregnancy can be tested to see if the fetus could be affected with the same disorder.

Which of the following is the most accurate statement regarding metabolic disease in the prenatal setting?

A. Fetuses affected with metabolic diseases are unlikely to come to term.
B. Knowing if a previously affected sibling of the mother was male or female helps determine risk in this and pregnancies.
C. Level 2 ultrasonography during the second trimester is likely to be helpful in detecting metabolic disease.
D. Poor fetal growth is common in metabolic diseases.
E. Prenatal metabolic screening is widely available.

334.

A 7-month-old boy presents to the emergency room lethargic and unarousable. Findings on physical examination are normal except for enlarged liver. Laboratory tests reveal a serum glucose concentration of 10.0 mg/dL. The mother tells you that the child slept through the night for the first time last night. Family history is negative for any serious or chronic illnesses. You are considering an inborn error of metabolism.

Which of the following is the most important lab test to order next?

    A. Serum calcium
    B. Serum ammonia
    C. Serum sodium
    D. Urine ketones
    E. Serum lactate

335.

You are evaluating a 2-day-old term infant because of abdominal distention. She fed normally the first day after birth but has had progressively increasing vomiting, which now is bilious. Physical examination demonstrates up-slanted palpebral fissures, a prominent tongue, and mild hypotonia. Upon passage of a nasogastric tube, you aspirate 80 mL of green-yellow material from her stomach. Abdominal radiographs, including a left lateral decubitus film, reveal dilated loops of bowel and air-fluid levels but no evidence of pneumatosis.

Which of the following is <u>least</u> likely to be found on history or physical exam?

    A. Advanced maternal age
    B. Heart murmur
    C. Hemihypertrophy
    D. Brushfield spots
    E. Transverse palmar crease

336.

As part of an ongoing evaluation for short stature associated with primary amenorrhea, a 15-year-old girl is noted to have streaked gonads during an abdominal and pelvic ultrasound examination.

Which of the following is the most commonly associated abnormality found on echocardiogram in patients with these clinical findings?

    A. Bicuspid aortic valves
    B. Mitral valve stenosis
    C. Pulmonary valve stenosis
    D. Dilation of the aortic root
    E. Atrial septal defect

337.

A 14-year-old male is referred for evaluation of possible Marfan syndrome. He has a history of mental retardation. He is noted to be above the 99th percentile for height and at the 10th percentile for weight. His limbs are elongated. He also has scoliosis and pectus excavatum.

Which of the following metabolic disorders have clinical features that often resemble Marfan syndrome?

A. Homocystinuria
B. Phenylketonuria
C. Maple syrup urine disease
D. Galactosemia
E. Carnitine deficiency

338.

During a well-child examination, a 3-week-old male is noted to have a loud, harsh, holosystolic murmur heard best at the left lower sternal border. His blood pressure is 75/40 in the right upper extremity and 70/38 in the right lower extremity. The femoral pulses are easily palpated. Due to the murmur, a chest x-ray is obtained that reveals an absent thymic shadow. Chromosome studies reveal microdeletions in chromosome 22.

Which of the following is most likely to be identified in other patients with this disorder?

A. Esophageal atresia
B. Congenital cataract
C. Splenomegaly and icteric sclera
D. An absent radius
E. Macrocephaly

339.

A 16-month-old boy is referred for developmental delay. His mother's pregnancy was uncomplicated. Delivery was unremarkable; birth weight was 7 pounds, 6 ounces. His current weight and height are both at the 97th percentile. Head circumference is at the 75th percentile. Facial features appear coarse. His forehead is prominent with associated hypertelorism. The abdomen is protuberant with both the liver and spleen enlarged. A family history reveals that several maternal uncles and a maternal great uncle have a facial appearance similar to the patient's and also have large heads and protruding abdomens.

Which of the following complications is most likely to occur as this patient grows older?

A. Renal failure
B. Recurrent spontaneous fractures of the long bones
C. Hepatocellular carcinoma
D. Acute myelogenous leukemia
E. Cardiac valvular leaflet dysfunction

340.

The parents of a 2-month-old boy are convinced that "there is something terribly wrong" with their son. Soon after the onset of most every feeding, he "screams out in pain." The parents also report that during bathing they have noticed that "some of his bones seem tender and even swollen." On physical exam the patient is irritable and febrile. There is a tender, firm swelling along the left mandible, which appears to make feeding difficult. A second firm, tender swelling is evident over the distal portion of the left femur. A skeletal survey to evaluate for non-accidental trauma reveals cortical thickening and periosteal new bone formation along the left mandible and distal portion of the left femur.

Which of the following statements is correct regarding patients with these findings?

A. Findings are consistent with and specific for non-accidental trauma.
B. Chronic renal failure typically develops by the 3rd-to-4th decade of life.
C. Recurrent episodes of osteomyelitis due to *S. aureus* are a common complication.
D. As a result of frequent pathological fractures, most patients are non-ambulatory by the 2nd decade of life.
E. Symptoms will likely resolve by 24–30 months of age.

341.

During a routine well-child visit a 5-year-old boy is discovered to have hearing loss. He has had two episodes of otitis media in the past. His older brother and grandfather also have a history of hearing loss. In addition, both siblings and their grandfather have a history of microscopic hematuria.

Which of the following complications is most likely to occur in this patient?

A. Recurrent urinary tract infections
B. Severe postural hypotension associated with urinary sodium loss
C. Recurrent episodes of gross hematuria
D. Recurrent fractures due to progressive osteoporosis
E. Macular degeneration

342.

A 2-week-old female is noted to have several distinct areas of grouped vesicles on her right lower extremity. Associated bullous lesions are also noted. In addition verrucous (wart-like) lesions are present along the dorsum of the right foot and surrounding the left ankle. During biopsy of a vesicular lesion, fluid is obtained for Wright's staining. The stain is negative for multinucleated giant cells, while the biopsy reveals inflammatory changes associated with eosinophils.

Which of the following best describes the prognosis in patients with this disorder?

A. Without a kidney transplant, most patients do not survive beyond adolescence.
B. Patients are at increased risk of central nervous system tumors.
C. Patients continue to develop verrucous lesions throughout childhood.
D. Growth is often markedly delayed due to associated pancreatic insufficiency.
E. Most patients have associated dental, hair, and nail abnormalities.

343.

A 3-year-old girl with a history of a seizure disorder is referred for evaluation of developmental delay. Her birth history is unremarkable. Her weight and height are at the 45th percentile; head circumference is at the 35th percentile. She is easily distracted and excitable—sometimes to the point that she will flap her hands while laughing. Although she is comfortable with her parents and interacts well with them, she exhibits little use of verbal language. She has a flattened occiput and keeps her mouth open, frequently drooling and thrusting out her tongue. On neurological exam there is evidence of increased tone, tremulous movements of the limbs, and ataxia.

Which of the following findings upon chromosome analysis is most likely to be identified in this patient?

A. Trisomy 21
B. Deletion of a gene segment on chromosome 15
C. Absence of one X chromosome
D. Reciprocal translocation between chromosome 9 and 22
E. Chromosome 21 mosaicism

344.

A 4-month-old girl presents with a 6-week history of a rash, poor feeding, frequent loose stools, and irritability. She is less interactive with her parents, smiling only occasionally. She breastfed well and gained weight appropriately during the first 2 months of life, at which time her feedings were changed to a cow's milk-based infant formula. Her weight has decreased from the 70th to the 35th percentile. On exam she appears ill. Her conjunctivas are injected. Multiple moist erythematous lesions, some with associated bullae and crusting, are present around her mouth, nose, and in the perineum. Eczematous patches of skin are present on both her feet and hands.

Which of the following is the likely cause of this patient's symptoms?

A. Severe combined immunodeficiency
B. Pancreatic insufficiency
C. Protein losing enteropathy
D. Guttate psoriasis
E. Zinc deficiency

345.

A 6-month-old boy presents for his first evaluation following birth after his mother fled from his abusive father and entered a shelter. Reportedly the boy's father refused to allow his mother to leave the home even for routine pediatric care. He takes a cow's milk-based infant formula and reportedly feeds well. However, his mother reports a history of frequent vomiting. She also describes two previous episodes consistent with generalized seizure activity. On examination his weight is below the 3rd percentile. He is not able to roll over and has poor head control. His mother also reports that his wet diapers "always smell musty."

Which of the following findings is most likely to be identified upon further evaluation of this patient?

    A. Elevated serum levels of phenylalanine
    B. Hyperammonemia
    C. Elevated serum levels of alloisoleucine
    D. Elevated serum levels of homogentisic acid
    E. Hyperuricemia

346.

A 4-month-old boy with a history of peripheral pulmonic stenosis presents for a follow-up health maintenance examination after he was noted to be gaining weight poorly during a previous visit 1 month earlier. His weight is below the 3rd percentile, and he is noted to be jaundiced. Laboratory results include evidence of direct hyperbilirubinemia and elevated serum aminotransferases. Review of a previous chest x-ray reveals the presence of several "butterfly vertebrae."

Which of the following is most likely to be identified during additional evaluation of this patient?

    A. Reduced number of interlobular bile ducts on percutaneous liver biopsy
    B. Choledochal cyst on abdominal ultrasound
    C. Inflammation consistent with neonatal hepatitis on percutaneous liver biopsy
    D. Complete deficiency of galactose-1-phosphate uridyl transferase (GALT)
    E. Absence of the gall bladder on abdominal ultrasound

347.

A 14-year-old mentally retarded boy recently diagnosed with Marfan syndrome presents to the emergency room after being found on the bathroom floor at school. When evaluated in the emergency room, it becomes clear that he has had a stroke. He is admitted to the intensive care unit.

Which of the following findings would provide the best evidence that the diagnosis of Marfan syndrome was incorrect?

    A. Elevated levels of serum ammonia
    B. Absence of the corpus callosum on head CT
    C. High arched palate associated with a bifid uvula
    D. Prolonged PT/PTT/Bleeding Time
    E. Elevated serum and urine levels of homocysteine

348.

The parents of a 5-year-old boy with trisomy 21 ask that a permission form be completed for their son to participate in the Special Olympics.

Which of the following represents a contraindication to participating in athletic events included in Special Olympics programs?

A. A history of frequent loss of bowel and bladder control associated with evidence of gait abnormality on physical exam
B. Hypothyroidism requiring treatment with $\geq$ 2mcg/kg of levothyroxine
C. BMI $\geq 95^{th}$ percentile
D. Ventricular septal defect involving the membranous septum
E. History of transient leukemia (transient myeloproliferative disorder)

349.

A 10-day-old girl is noted to have 22% blast (megakaryoblasts) forms in the peripheral blood during laboratory evaluation for jaundice. She is otherwise asymptomatic with the exception of scattered vesiculopustular lesions. The percentage of blasts in the bone marrow is lower than that in the peripheral blood.

During additional cytogenetic studies, which of the following chromosomal abnormalities is most likely to be identified in this patient?

A. 45,X
B. 47,XX + 21
C. 47,XX + 13
D. 47,XX + 18
E. 47,XXX

350.

A 4-year-old boy presents for an initial health maintenance examination after being adopted from Guatemala. On physical examination, he is noted to have a short neck, low hair line, and limited range of motion of his head and neck. Anteroposterior, lateral, and oblique views of the cervical spine show evidence of multiple fused cervical vertebrae.

Which of the following congenital orthopedic abnormalities is a commonly associated finding in patients with this disorder?

A. Absent radius
B. Failure of the scapula to descend to its normal position
C. Developmental dysplasia of the hip
D. Genu varum
E. Talipes equinovarus

351.

During a health maintenance visit a 4-month-old female is noted to have a skull deformity due to premature fusion of both coronal and one sagittal sutures.

Which of the following additional findings on physical examination would indicate that this patient's cranial abnormalities are consistent with Apert, rather than Crouzon, syndrome?

A. Leg length discrepancy
B. Prominent ocular proptosis
C. Congenital stenosis or atresia of the external ear canals
D. Occipital plagiocephaly
E. Syndactyly of the 2nd, 3rd, and 4th fingers and toes

352.

During a health maintenance visit a 4-year-old girl is noted to be at the 5th percentile for height and at the 55th percentile for weight. Findings on physical examination include a webbed neck, broad forehead, hypertelorism, pectus excavatum, and cubitus valgus. A prominent pulmonic ejection click, heard best at the left upper sternal border, is present immediately after the first heart sound heard. The second heart sound is spit and a short II/VI medium-pitched systolic ejection murmur is present.

Which of the following karyotypes is most likely to be identified during additional evaluation of this patient?

A. 46,XX
B. 45,X
C. 45,X/46, XX
D. 45,X/46, XY
E. 47,XXX

353.

A CT scan of the head in a 2-year-old girl with a history of developmental delay and seizures shows evidence of unilateral intracranial calcification in the occipitoparietal region and underlying atrophy of the ipsilateral cerebral hemisphere. A plain skull radiograph reveals that the intracranial calcifications have a serpentine-like appearance.

Which of the following is likely to be identified on physical examination in this patient?

A. A hypomelanotic macule on the trunk
B. A roughened raised lesion with an "orange-peel" consistency in the lumbosacral region
C. Multiple hyperpigmented 2–3 mm macules in the axilla
D. A unilateral facial nevus involving the upper face and eyelid
E. Multiple angiomas located in the peripheral portions of the retina

354.

As part of a diagnostic workup for hypotonia, a 10-day-old male born at term via caesarean section is found to have a chromosome 15q partial deletion. Associated findings include a diminished cry, poor suck reflex, and decreased activity. At times the patient has required tube feedings. Several dysmorphic features are evident on physical examination, including dolichocephaly, "almond-shaped" eyes, and a small-appearing mouth and thin upper lip. The testes are undescended, and the penis appears small.

As this patient grows older, which of the following is most likely to occur?

    A. Morbid obesity
    B. Tall stature for genetic background
    C. Chronic renal failure
    D. Inflammatory bowel disease
    E. Recurrent fractures following minor trauma

355.

Upon initial examination in the newborn nursery, a term female infant weighing 3.6 kg is noted to have a murmur. An echocardiogram shows narrowing of the right ventricular outflow tract and an overriding aorta associated with a ventricular septal defect and right ventricular hypertrophy. Plain radiographs of the right and left forearms reveal bilateral absence of the radii.

Which of the following is most likely to be identified upon further evaluation of this patient?

    A. Bilateral cataracts and microphthalmia
    B. Marked decrease in megakaryocytes on bone marrow examination
    C. Hepatosplenomegaly
    D. Extensive blistering of the fingers, hands and feet
    E. Hypocalcemia

356.

A woman at 37 weeks gestation is admitted for a planned cesarean section. She has been closely followed throughout her pregnancy because of multiple fetal anomalies noted on prenatal ultrasound, including cleft lip/palate, polycystic kidneys, absence of the corpus callosum, enlarged ventricles, ventricular septal defect and polydactyly. A viable male infant, weighing 2.9 kg, is delivered and transferred to the neonatal intensive care unit. Physical examination findings include several focal sharply demarcated ulcerated plaques on the scalp, which are absent of skin and covered only by a tense membrane.

Which of the following karyotypes is most likely to be identified upon further evaluation of this patient?

    A. 47,XY, + 18
    B. 47,XY, + 21
    C. 47,XY, +13
    D. 47,XXY
    E. 46,XY/47, XY + 18

357.

Following an emergency cesarean section due to fetal distress, a 36-week gestation male is placed on a ventilator due to respiratory distress. His mother had a history of oligohydramnios during her pregnancy. He is noted to have significant laxity of the abdominal musculature, scoliosis, and easily palpable bilaterally enlarged kidneys.

Which of the following associated findings is likely to be identified upon further evaluation of this patient?

A. Abdominal cryptorchidism
B. Congenital cataracts
C. Absent corpus callosum
D. Biliary atresia
E. Absent radius

358.

A 1-day-old male infant is noted to have difficulty feeding due to micrognathia. A chest x-ray, obtained due to concern about possible aspiration after an episode of choking during attempts to feed, reveals an absent thymus. Soon after the x-ray is obtained, he is noted to have generalized tonic clonic seizure activity. The patient is subsequently transferred to the neonatal intensive care unit, where additional evaluation includes an electrocardiogram.

Which of the following findings is most likely to be identified upon review of the electrocardiogram?

A. A shortened QTc interval
B. ST segment elevation
C. Peaked T waves
D. Prolonged PR interval
E. Type 1 second-degree heart block (Wenckebach phenomenon)

359.

A 7-year-old boy with a history of attention deficit disorder presents for evaluation because his parents are concerned that he is "overmedicated." He has been taking an extended preparation of methylphenidate (36 mg) for the previous 4 months because of impulsive behavior, outbursts of aggression, and difficulty staying on task. Over the last week he has, at times, been "walking like he is drunk" and had difficulty maintaining his balance and climbing stairs. Also, his parents were recently contacted by his teacher because of "slurred speech and poor handwriting." On physical examination he is visibly upset, refuses to follow simple commands, and is slurring his words. His gait is ataxic. Additional findings include increased deep tendon reflexes in the lower extremities, bilateral ankle clonus, and hyperpigmentation in the axilla and over the knees and elbows.

Which of the following tests is most likely to be abnormal upon further evaluation of this patient?

A. Levels of serum ceruloplasmin
B. Levels of serum triglycerides, cholesterol, and phospholipids
C. Levels of serum creatinine kinase, aspartate aminotransferase, and lactate dehydrogenase
D. Levels of glycosaminoglycans in the urine
E. Levels of plasma very long chain fatty acids

360.

A mother brings her 1-month-old white male to clinic because he has seemed "weak" over the last several days. He doesn't feed as well as normal, and his breathing seems "different." He's had no fever and no illness. He spits up a little after each feeding. He was born at term without complications to a gravida 1 mother. He went home 2 days after birth and was given a healthy report at his newborn visit when he was a week old.

On physical examination he appears alert but hypotonic and keeps his mouth open. Heart sounds are normal but with a slightly increased rate. Liver is below the right costal margin approximately 3–4 cm. Pulses are normal.

CXR shows an enlarged heart.
EKG shows increased QRS complexes and shortened PR intervals.

Glucose level in office—87 (last bottle was 3–4 hours ago).

Which of the following is the most likely diagnosis?

- A. Glycogen storage disease Type Ia (von Gierke disease)
- B. Glycogen storage disease Type IIa (Pompe disease)
- C. Spinal muscular atrophy
- D. Hurler syndrome
- E. Muscular dystrophy

361.

You are seeing a 3-year-old male for the first time. He is very friendly and outgoing. Mentally he is well below average. He is at the 15th percentile for weight and 5th percentile for height. He has short palpebral fissures with depressed nasal bridge, long philtrum, and prominent lips with open mouth. He has a hoarse voice and a low-pitched, rough, ejection systolic murmur heard best at the sternal edge of the second intercostal space. You also feel a thrill in the suprasternal notch. No webbing of the neck. He also has short nails.

Which of the following is the most likely diagnosis?

- A. Noonan syndrome
- B. Kabuki syndrome
- C. Smith-Lemli-Opitz syndrome
- D. Williams syndrome
- E. Costello syndrome

362.

A full-term infant is born to a 42-year-old G2P2 female with a normal prenatal course. The infant vomits the first feeding of dextrose water and proceeds with emesis of all feeds over the ensuing 24 hours. Some of the bouts of emesis are notably greenish-yellow in color. Physical examination reveals a crying child with a heart rate of 210 bpm, a protruding tongue, a non-distended abdomen without hepatosplenomegaly, mild hypotonia, and a patent anus. Plain films of the abdomen reveal a "double bubble sign."

Further neonatal evaluation should include all of the following <u>except</u>:

A. Chromosomal evaluation
B. Evaluation of the adrenal axis
C. Thyroid function testing
D. Echocardiography
E. CBC with peripheral smear evaluation

363.

You are called to a cesarean section delivery of a 41-year-old G1P0 female for her failure to progress. She has a history of Crohn Disease. She is visiting your city over the Christmas holidays and has received all of her prenatal care in another state. She currently takes only a prenatal vitamin and reports no flares of inflammatory bowel disease in the last 8 months. A female infant is born with a cleft lip and palate and significant respiratory distress. The infant is successfully resuscitated with intubation and is transferred to the NICU.

Physical examination reveals low-set malformed ears, a prominent occiput, rocker-bottom feet, clenched hands with overlapping fingers, nail hypoplasia, a heart murmur, and hypotonia. Chromosomal analysis reveals normal chromosomes.

Which of the following is the most likely etiology of the infant's abnormal phenotype?

A. Perinatal exposure to sulfasalazine during the 1st trimester
B. A single gene dominant mutation
C. 200 linear CGG repeats located at Xq27.3
D. Perinatal exposure to methotrexate
E. A DNA rearrangement in the chromosomal area 21q22.2-22.3

364.

A mother and her 17-year-old daughter present to your office to discuss contraceptive options for the adolescent. The patient's past medical history is significant only for normal childhood illnesses. She is in the 11th grade and averages Bs and Cs in school. She takes no medication and has no allergies. She began menstruating at age 13 with cycles lasting 5–7 days in duration. She has never been sexually active.

PHYSICAL EXAMINATION:

BP 152/86 HR 87 T 98.6° RR 16
Height 4′9″ (maternal height 5′4″, paternal height 5′9″) Weight 117 lbs.

Significant findings: Grade 2/6 systolic murmur maximal at the left upper sternal border without radiation, 1+ pitting edema to the knees bilaterally, Tanner stage 4-5/5 with widely spaced nipples.

Which of the following is most appropriate?

A. Full chromosomal analysis and echocardiography.
B. No contraception is necessary. She has Turner syndrome and is likely infertile.
C. Initiation of diuretic therapy for the elevated blood pressure prior to initiating therapy with oral contraceptive pills.

   D. Begin therapy with oral contraceptive pills. Have the patient return on 2 more occasions for blood
       pressure determinations before initiating therapy for hypertension.

   E. Send a buccal smear sample for sex chromatin evaluation.

365.

You are called to the newborn nursery to evaluate a full-term infant with abnormal facies. The mother is a 24-year-old G1P1 with no prenatal care, who presented to the labor unit after 6 hours of contractions with intact membranes and normal vital signs. The male infant was delivered vaginally without complications, but the nurses notice the infant is small with a "low-set jaw." Physical examination reveals a small-for-gestational-age infant, micrognathia, posteriorly rotated and low-set ears, epicanthal folds, simian creases of the palms, and syndactyly of the 2nd and 3rd toes. A hazy appearance of the right cornea is notable when evaluating the red reflexes. Muscular tone is decreased, and the infant sucks and swallows poorly with a trial of dextrose water by nipple.

Which of the following is true?

   A. The infant has clinical features suggestive of trisomy 18 and may have concomitant rocker-bottom feet, hypoplasia of nail beds, and normal intelligence.

   B. The infant has clinical features suggestive of Down syndrome and may have concomitant congenital heart disease, thyroid disease, and mental retardation.

   C. The infant has clinical features suggestive of Noonan syndrome and may have concomitant sterility, an undescended testis, and normal intelligence.

   D. The infant has clinical features suggestive of Smith-Lemli-Opitz syndrome and may have concomitant hypospadias, congenital heart disease, and death by 18 months of age.

   E. The infant has clinical features suggestive of trisomy 2 and may have concomitant mental retardation and heart disease.

366.

The mother of a 4-day-old male infant brings the baby to you with complaints of 4 episodes of non-bilious emesis today. The last 2 episodes were projectile in character. The pregnancy and delivery were normal for this term infant. He experienced frequent spit-ups from birth but was discharged on day 2 of life. On physical examination, he appears alert. His respiratory rate is 60, and his pulse rate is 160. His anterior fontanel is slightly sunken. His mucous membranes are dry. The remainder of his exam is normal. His CBC is normal. His serum ammonia level is elevated, but his serum pH and bicarbonate levels are normal.

Which of the following do you suspect as the etiology of this infant's signs and symptoms?

   A. Urea cycle defect
   B. Sepsis
   C. Serum organic acidemia
   D. Pyloric stenosis
   E. Serum amino acidemia

367.

A 1-month-old is brought to you for evaluation. He has had a clear runny nose without fever for about
3 days. Today, the mother noticed that he was irritable, less active than normal, and "breathing funny." She had a normal pregnancy and delivery. On physical examination, he is awake but motionless. He is tachypneic and

tachycardic but afebrile and normotensive. He has some clear rhinorrhea. A bittersweet aroma can be detected from the child. The remainder of his exam is normal. His metabolic profile reveals a high anion gap acidosis with hypoglycemia and ketosis.

Which of the following is the most likely diagnosis?

A. Sepsis
B. Meningitis
C. Intermittent maple syrup urine disease
D. Urea cycle defect
E. None of the answers is likely

368.

A 3-month-old, who was born at term and had a non-eventful pregnancy and birth, is brought to you for lethargy and bloody stools. The child was in his normal state until yesterday, when the mother noted increasing amounts of blood in his stools. This morning, she had difficulty arousing him. He drank his bottle with some improvement, but is now getting lethargic again. On physical examination, he is tachypneic, tachycardic, and afebrile. He has a full anterior fontanel. His liver is moderately enlarged, causing his abdomen to protrude. During your examination, the child has a sustained tonic-clonic seizure.

Which of the following is the most appropriate to administer now?

A. Intramuscular administration of glucagon
B. Intravenous administration of a glucose-containing solution
C. Intravenous administration of 3% NaCl
D. Intravenous administration of fosphenytoin sodium
E. Intravenous administration of calcium gluconate

369.

A 16-month-old female is brought to the emergency room with generalized tonic-clonic seizures. For the past 3 days, she has been vomiting and had several episodes of diarrhea. She has been tolerating some liquids, but has refused all solids. This morning, her parents found her unresponsive with tonic-clonic movement of her extremities. Physical examination reveals an unresponsive toddler. She is tachypneic and tachycardic. She is afebrile. The anterior fontanelle is closed. The liver is moderately enlarged and smooth. The remainder of the exam is normal. A complete metabolic panel reveals a normal anion gap acidosis with glucose of 18 mg/dL. Her AST and ALT are three times normal. Her CBC and urinalysis are normal, without ketones present. A CT of the head is normal. CSF cell counts and protein are within normal limits. You infuse a dextrose solution and start ceftriaxone. The child's glucose normalizes, but improvement in her mental status is very slow and the acidosis persists. Serum organic acids are ordered, but the results will not be available for 1 week.

Which of the following do you consider?

A. Broader antibiotic coverage
B. Biotin administration
C. Administration of carnitine
D. Thiamine administration
E. Exchange transfusion

GROWTH and DEVELOPMENT

370.

At 11:45 a.m., the last visit before your afternoon off, you have a "new patient" visit. Ms. Andrews has brought her 7-month-old son to see you. She has just moved back in with her parents due to a very messy divorce. One of the major conflict points in their marriage was the husband's belief that children did not need medical care of any sort. She had been concerned about her son's development, but his father would not let her bring him to see anyone for evaluation. Your history and physical examination reveals the following:

PRENATAL HISTORY: No prenatal care history; mother states she smoked and had an occasional drink of ETOH during her pregnancy.

BIRTH HISTORY: Normal spontaneous vaginal delivery at term at home with a neighbor acting as a midwife; birth weight was approximately 3 kg; no other information available.

HOSPITALIZATIONS AND SURGERIES: None
MEDICATIONS: None
IMMUNIZATIONS: None

DIET: Breast milk ad lib with the addition of jar baby food (fruits, vegetables).

FAMILY HISTORY: No developmental problems or mental retardation.

SOCIAL HISTORY: Mother and father are going through a divorce, and mother recently moved back home; she is currently unemployed.

REVIEW OF SYSTEMS: No other problems noted.

PHYSICAL EXAMINATION:
    Weight: 7 kg (5%)   Length: 66 cm (10%)   Head circumference: 41 (5%)
    Heart rate: 92   Respiratory rate: 20   Temperature: 98.6° F

    HEENT: Normal
    Chest: Clear to auscultation
    Heart: Regular rate and rhythm
    Abdomen: Soft bowel sounds present, no hepatosplenomegaly or masses
    Genitalia: Normal male with bilateral descended testes
    Skin: Normal
    Neuro: Cranial nerves 2–12 were intact, normal tone, nonfocal

DEVELOPMENTAL: Lifts his head and chest in almost a vertical axis; he has no head lag when pulled to a sitting position and can hold his head steady. He does not roll over. He seems to enjoy sitting with full truncal support. When held erect he pushes with his feet. He holds his hands in midline and reaches, grasps objects, and brings them to his mouth. When he sees a pellet, he makes no move toward it. He laughs aloud and becomes excited at the sight of food.

Which of the following would you tell her?

A. Her son has the developmental age of approximately 4 months.
B. Her son's development is normal for a 7-month-old.
C. Her son has the developmental age of approximately 3 months.
D. Her son has the developmental age of approximately 10 months.
E. There is a wide variation in developmental milestones and his minor delays will correct themselves.

371.

Mrs. Obudala presents to your clinic for a 2-month health supervision examination of her infant. The mother states that her daughter has been growing well, but she is worried about her development. When pressed further about her concerns, she starts to cry. Mrs. Obudala had a sister who was severely mentally retarded, and she remembers that her mother knew something was different about that child by 2 months of age. Mrs. Obudala is concerned because she has no other children and really cannot tell if her daughter is developing normally. The remainder of your history and physical examination reveals the following:

PRENATAL HISTORY: Started at 8 weeks of gestation; mother had a febrile episode at 4-months gestation, otherwise unremarkable. She denies tobacco or ETOH consumption during pregnancy.

BIRTH HISTORY: The infant was born at 36 weeks with a birthweight of 3.1 kg by cesarean delivery for failure to progress. Mother's membranes were ruptured at the time of delivery. Mother states the baby's APGAR scores were 8 and 9.

HOSPITALIZATIONS: None
SURGERY: None
MEDICATIONS: Liquid multivitamin once a day
IMMUNIZATIONS: Hepatitis B #1 after delivery in the hospital
ALLERGIES: None

DIET: Breastfeeding; infant feeds approximately 15–20 minutes on each breast every 2–3 hours.

FAMILY HISTORY: Mom and dad are both healthy; no other children.

SOCIAL HISTORY: Dad is a chemical engineer, mother is an accountant.

REVIEW OF SYSTEMS: Negative for 10 systems.

PHYSICAL EXAMINATION:
Weight: 4.5 kg (50%)   Length: 55 cm (50%)   Head circumference: 38.8 cm (50%);
Heart rate: 123   Respirations: 22   Temperature: 37.6° C (99.6° F)

HEENT: Red reflex present bilaterally
Chest: Clear to auscultation
Heart: Regular rate and rhythm without murmurs
Abdomen: Soft with no hepatosplenomegaly, no masses
Genitalia: Normal female
Skin: Normal
Neuro: Cranial nerves 2–12 grossly intact, normal tone, reflexes bilateral

DEVELOPMENT: Raises her head slightly, with her head sustained in the same plane as the body on vertical suspension; head lags on pulling to sitting position; follows a red ball about 180°; smiles to social contact and will listen to the voice of the examiner and coos.

Which of the following do you tell the mother?

    A. Her infant has the developmental milestones of a newborn.
    B. Her infant has the developmental milestones of a 4-week-old.
    C. Her infant has normal developmental milestones for an 8-week-old.
    D. Her infant has significant developmental delay.
    E. Her infant has advanced development.

372.

You are working in the afterhours clinic during a typical January evening. In the four hours you have been there, you have seen 32 patients and you are ready for your night to be finished. You find that the last appointment is one of your partner's patients who has been lost to follow-up. Your partner has sent a certified letter to their last known address letting them know they have missed their last two health supervision visits, and that she was concerned about the fact that the child was not developing appropriately. Your partner further stated that if they did not come to see her soon, she was going to alert the authorities and start pursuing the situation as a neglect case. The nurse informs you that the mother received the certified letter today and immediately made an appointment, because she was furious she had received such a letter and wanted to let "someone know about it." As you walk in the room, you note that the patient is a 1-year-old male named Samuel. As you enter the room, you note Samuel is sitting alone while his mother is pacing the examination room. She tells you quite confidently there is nothing wrong with her son. After you calm the mother down, you obtain the following past medical history.

PRENATAL HISTORY: Prenatal history care at 5 months, no tobacco or ETOH consumption.
NATAL HISTORY: Normal spontaneous vaginal delivery with a birth weight of 3.4 kg.

HOSPITALIZATIONS: Group B streptococcal meningitis at 3 weeks of age; patient was on the ventilator for 2 weeks and required "medications for blood pressure" for approximately 10 days. Mother states she was told the computed tomography of his head was not normal but did not know what the abnormality was.

SURGERY: Had a central venous catheter placed for intravenous treatment of the group B streptococcal meningitis.

ALLERGIES: None
MEDICATIONS: None
IMMUNIZATIONS: Last shots at 6 months

DIET: Just transitioned to whole cow's milk, also eating table foods

FAMILY HISTORY: No developmental problems in the family; the father, however, was in "resource classes" for middle and high school. Has a 4-year-old sister who is alive and well.

SOCIAL HISTORY: Dad is disabled and mother works in the school cafeteria.
REVIEW OF SYSTEMS: Normal hearing screen after the meningitis, otherwise negative

PHYSICAL EXAMINATION:

Weight: 11 kg (75%) Length: 76 cm (75%) Head circumference: 44 cm (< 5%)

Heart rate: 84 Respiratory rate: 18 Temperature: 37.5° C (99.5° F)

HEENT:	Microcephalic but otherwise normal
Chest:	Clear to auscultation, scar on his left upper chest from the central line
Heart:	Regular rate and rhythm without murmurs
Abdomen:	Soft with positive bowel sounds, no hepatosplenomegaly, no masses
Genitalia:	Normal male with bilateral descended testes; Skin: normal
Neuro:	Cranial nerves 2–12 were grossly intact, normal tone, reflexes present and equal bilaterally, toes downgoing bilaterally

DEVELOPMENTAL: Sits alone without support indefinitely, pulls to standing position and will walk holding onto the furniture in the examination room—but cannot walk independently; grasps objects with his thumb and forefinger, but does not release objects to examiner upon request; uncovers a hidden toy and attempts to recover it when it is dropped. Demonstrates repetitive consonant sounds (e.g., mama, dada) but knows no other words, will respond to his name, waves "bye-bye" but will not play a simple ball game.

Which of the following do you tell the mother about Samuel?

A. Her son is developing appropriately.
B. Her son will probably be in resource classes like his father.
C. Her son has a developmental age of a 6-month-old.
D. Her son has a developmental age of a 9-month-old.
E. Any abnormality in development can be attributed to the meningitis.

373.

Which of the following is a correct method to calculate mid-parental height (using inches) for a girl?

A. (Mother's Height + Father's Height)/2
B. (Mother's Height + 5 + Father's Height)/2
C. (Father's Height – 5 + Mother's Height)/2
D. [(Mother's Height + Father's Height) – 5]/2
E. (Mother's Height – 5 + Father's Height)/2

374.

The Martinez family has just returned from a three-year missionary trip to Africa. They are excited to introduce you to their 2-year-old daughter Elizabeth. You are familiar with the Martinez family because you cared for their other two children prior to their stay in Africa. Elizabeth was born in Africa, and this is the first time you have examined her. After you speak to the family a bit, Mrs. Martinez asks if she could use the phone in your office. The question catches you off guard but you say, sure, and lead her out of the room. Once outside, she stops you and explains she did not want to talk in front of the other children or Elizabeth. She tells you she is worried about Elizabeth's development. She has seemed "slow" to do things as compared to the other two children. You obtain the following history:

PRENATAL HISTORY: Followed by a physician starting at 3-months gestation, had some gestational diabetes but was controlled with diet; otherwise, she states the pregnancy was normal.

NATAL HISTORY: Born in the clinic in Africa after a long labor. She labored approximately 22 hours and required a forceps delivery. Elizabeth had required vigorous stimulation after delivery and some blow-by oxygen.

HOSPITALIZATIONS: None
SURGERY: None
IMMUNIZATIONS: Has not received the varicella vaccine; otherwise, "up to date"
ALLERGIES: None

FAMILY HISTORY: Dad is a minister; mother is a housewife, both siblings alive and well

SOCIAL HISTORY: Will be living in the United States for at least 5 years until the next overseas assignment becomes available

DEVELOPMENTAL HISTORY:
Sat by herself at 10 months, walked at 14 months, babbled at 9 months

REVIEW OF SYSTEMS: No head trauma, did break her arm at 15 months but otherwise the review of systems is negative

PHYSICAL EXAMINATION:
Weight: 12 Kg (50%)   Length: 86 cm (50%)   Head circumference: 49 cm (50%)
Heart rate: 88   Respiratory rate: 18   Temperature: 37.7° C (99.8° F)

HEENT: Scarred tympanic membrane on the right
Chest: Clear to auscultation
Heart: Regular rate and rhythm without murmurs, clicks, or rubs
Abdomen: Soft with bowel sounds present, no hepatosplenomegaly, no masses
Genitalia: Normal female external genitalia
Neuro: Cranial nerves 2–12 were grossly intact, reflexes were bilateral and intact although the lower extremities were 3+ and the upper extremities were 1+. No sustained clonus was demonstrated, and the toes were downgoing bilaterally. Her lower extremities demonstrated increased tone as compared to the upper extremities; her gait was normal

DEVELOPMENTAL: She could walk alone but had to crawl up stairs. She could make a tower of 3 cubes, make a line with a crayon, and insert a pellet into a bottle. She could follow simple commands and could name simple objects (e.g., ball). She indicates her desires by pointing.

Which of the following statements do you tell Mrs. Martinez about Elizabeth?

A. She has the developmental age of 18 months.
B. She has the developmental age of 15 months.
C. She has the developmental age of 24 months.
D. She has the developmental age of 30 months.
E. She suffered birth asphyxia and is mentally retarded.

375.

You are just about to finish a shift in the emergency room when local police officers bring in a little girl they have found wandering in a local city park. The police do not know her name or even how old she is. They have brought her to your emergency room to see if you can tell them about how old she is. There is no other history available to you. Her physical examination reveals the following:

Weight: 11.5 kg   Length: 82 cm   Head circumference: 47 cm
Heart rate: 92   Respiratory rate: 25   Temperature: 37.7° C (99.8° F)

HEENT:	Clear
Chest:	Clear to auscultation
Heart:	Regular rate and rhythm with no murmur, clicks or rubs
Abdomen:	Soft with positive bowel sounds, no masses, no hepatosplenomegaly
Extremities:	No cyanosis, clubbing or edema
Skin:	No rashes
Neuro:	Alert and oriented, cranial nerves 2–12 are grossly intact, all reflexes are 2+/4+ and bilateral, her tone is normal

DEVELOPMENTAL: She can run although her gait is somewhat stiff; she can walk up the stairs if you hold her hand; she can make a tower of 4 cubes and imitates scribbling; she can dump a pellet from a bottle. She speaks about 10 words and can identify one or more body parts; she can feed herself but still wears a diaper. She does complain when her diaper is dirty.

Which of the following do you tell the police officer, based upon her weight, head circumference, and her developmental examination?

   A. She is approximately 18 months of age.
   B. She is approximately 24 months of age.
   C. She is approximately 12 months of age.
   D. She is approximately 15 months of age.
   E. You cannot provide them with an approximate age.

376.

Your sister asks if you think your three-year-old nephew Adam is developing normally. There has been nothing that has happened to the child, but she works in a day care for handicapped children and is fearful for her own child. To help her with her fears, you tell her you will check him out for her. She reminds you of the following history:

PRENATAL HISTORY: Prenatal history care beginning at 2-months gestation, no illnesses during pregnancy; no tobacco or ETOH use

NATAL HISTORY: Normal spontaneous vaginal delivery with a birth weight of 4 kg, home in 24 hours

HOSPITALIZATIONS:	None
SURGERIES:	None
ALLERGIES:	None
IMMUNIZATIONS:	Up to date

MEDICATIONS: None
DIET: Normal table food, one chewable multivitamin/day

FAMILY HISTORY: No history of developmental or learning problems on either side of the family
SOCIAL HISTORY: Dad is a grocer, mom started working at the day care 5 months ago. Adam does attend daycare while mom and dad work.

REVIEW OF SYSTEMS: Negative for 10 systems

PHYSICAL EXAMINATION:
Weight: 16 kg (>75%)   Length:100 cm (> 75%)   Head circumference: 50 cm (75%)
Heart rate: 82   Respiratory rate: 21   Temperature: 37.7° C (99.8° F)

HEENT:	Clear
Chest:	Clear to auscultation
Heart:	Regular rate and rhythm with no murmur, clicks, or rubs
Abdomen:	Soft with positive bowel sounds, no masses, no hepatosplenomegaly
Extremities:	No cyanosis, clubbing, or edema
Genitalia:	Normal male with bilaterally descended testes
Skin:	No rashes
Neuro:	Alert and oriented, cranial nerves 2–12 are grossly intact, all reflexes are 2+/4+ and bilateral, tone and gait are normal

DEVELOPMENTAL EXAM: Can momentarily stand on one foot, copies a circle and can make a tower of 10 cubes. He knows his age and sex, can repeat 3 objects back to you, and plays simple games with the examiner. He can help in dressing himself and can wash his hands.

Which of the following do you tell your sister?

    A. Adam is developmentally delayed to approximately 24 months.
    B. Adam has the developmental age of 48 months.
    C. Adam will not be able to attend "normal classes."
    D. Adam should be removed from daycare.
    E. Adam's development is appropriate for his age.

377.

A mother of a 6-year-old boy presents with concerns about nightmares and night screaming in her son.

During which of the following stages of sleep do night terrors most commonly occur?

    A. Stage 1, non-REM sleep
    B. Stage 2, non-REM sleep
    C. Stage 3, non-REM sleep
    D. Stage 4, non-REM sleep
    E. REM sleep

378.

In discussing different items in a 5-year-old's health supervision visit, Mrs. Corleone admits that she is worried that her son Michael might not be ready for kindergarten this next fall. She is worried he will not be able to do his schoolwork because he has been sheltered all of his life and is "not very mature." She has 3 other children, but Michael has always been a "special child" since he is the youngest. The mother wants him to be able to perform well in school because she doesn't want him to follow his father and brothers into the family business; she wants him to "make something out of himself." You review the following pertinent points of his history:

PRENATAL HISTORY: Fourth pregnancy to a 30-year-old woman with good prenatal history care; there was a positive history of tobacco use by the father (only outside), but she did not smoke

NATAL HISTORY: Normal spontaneous vaginal delivery

HOSPITALIZATIONS:	None
SURGERY:	None
IMMUNIZATIONS:	Up to date
MEDICATIONS:	None
ALLERGIES:	None
FAMILY HISTORY:	No history of developmental or learning problems

SOCIAL HISTORY: Father is in the "olive oil business;" mother is a housewife and always accompanied by a bodyguard, who is a very large man that never says a word

REVIEW OF SYSTEMS: Negative for 10 systems

PHYSICAL EXAMINATION:
Weight: 19.8 kg (50%) Height: 107 cm (25%)
Heart rate: 76   Respiratory rate: 18   Temperature: 37.7° C (99.8° F)

HEENT:	Clear
Chest:	Clear to auscultation
Heart:	Regular rate and rhythm with no murmur, clicks or rubs
Abdomen:	Soft with positive bowel sounds, no masses, no hepatosplenomegaly
Extremities:	No cyanosis, clubbing, or edema
Genitalia:	Normal male with bilaterally descended testes
Skin:	No rashes
Neuro:	Alert and oriented, cranial nerves 2–12 are grossly intact, all reflexes are 2+/4+; bilateral tone and gait are normal

DEVELOPMENTAL EXAM:
Michael can skip, copy a triangle, name 4 colors, and count 10 pennies correctly. He dresses and undresses himself and asks questions about the meaning of words.

Which of the following should you tell his mother?

A. Michael is significantly delayed in his development.
B. Michael has been too sheltered in his life.
C. Michael has the appropriate developmental skills to attend kindergarten.
D. You cannot determine if Michael is ready for kindergarten at this visit.
E. Not to bring the body guard with her anymore.

379.

A mother brings her 9-month-old to see you for his well-child visit. She wants to know if he is on target developmentally.

He should be able to do all of the following <u>except</u>:

A. Walk independently
B. Pull to standing position
C. Creep or crawl
D. Use pincer grasp
E. Use repetitive sounds (mama, dada)

380.

A mother brings her 18-month-old in for his well-child exam. This is her first child, and she is very concerned about his development and is always comparing him to other children. You ask her several questions and assure her that he is doing just fine.

He should be able to do all of the following <u>except</u>:

A. Identify one or more body parts
B. Use 2- or 3-word sentences
C. Scribble
D. Run stiffly
E. Feed self

381.

A mother brings her 18-month-old daughter to see you for "passing out." She is very concerned and tells you this is the second time this has happened. On questioning her, you find out that both episodes started when the child got upset (once due to minor injury and once due to limit-setting). She then let out a couple of cries and with the last long cry, turned blue and passed out. With both episodes, she began breathing again within 30–60 seconds. On physical examination, the patient is active and happy. Growth is normal, BP 76/45, temperature 98.9°, HR 120, and physical examination is completely normal.

Which of the following do you recommend next?

A. Order an EEG.
B. Refer to a cardiologist.
C. Reassure her mother that attacks are harmless and will eventually resolve on their own.
D. Order electrolytes.
E. Tell the mother to give the child whatever she wants so she won't get mad.

382.

A 6-year-old boy presents for evaluation of repeated involuntary passage of stool into his underwear. He only has difficulties while awake and has not had any "accidents" while sleeping. A physical examination reveals no physical etiology for the fecal incontinence.

Which of the following is <u>not</u> correct with regard to his condition?

A. The child needs to sit on the toilet, preferably 2 times per day, for intervals of 5–10 minutes.
B. Soiling accidents are the responsibility of both the child and the parent, and they equally should be involved in the clean-up.
C. Some children are resistant to sitting due to fear of having a painful bowel movement.
D. A reward system that provides incentives for cooperating with a sitting schedule is helpful.
E. For the oppositional child, refusal to sit on the toilet should be met with a privilege restriction (for example, bedtime is moved up by the minutes allotted to toilet time).

383.

Which of the following is <u>not</u> true with regards to treatment of enuresis?

A. In an 8-year-old, a "potty alarm" should achieve 80% initial success rates.
B. Restriction of fluids 90 minutes to 120 minutes before bedtime is reasonable.
C. A technique known as "overcorrection" may be effective.
D. Use of a "potty alarm" is appropriate for children aged 4 years and above.
E. Pharmacologic therapy may be effective.

384.

Priscilla is a 14-month-old girl who started to place unusual, nonnutritive substances in her mouth. Her mother has noted that this process is increasing in frequency.

Which of the following is correct?

A. Pica is frequently associated with mental retardation.
B. It usually starts at 2 years of age.
C. In the case of potentially dangerous pica, use of mild punishment is never recommended (time-outs).
D. Dangerous items should not be removed from the child, but the child should be instructed to dispose of them.
E. It is best not to praise a child when she is exposed to potential agents and has refrained from placing them in her mouth.

385.

Lauren Cross is a 10-year-old child who has frequent temper tantrums. Sometimes her parents can't figure out how a "lovely child" turns into a "holy terror" in less than a minute. Any little thing can set her off.

Which of the following is true with regard to "time-out" as a tool for reducing temper tantrums?

A. Time-out is instinctive for children.
B. A warning that a time-out is coming is usually effective.
C. Time-out has lost its usefulness when a child says that she does not mind or even likes time-outs.
D. After a time-out, it is best to remind the child of the incident to prevent further occurrences.
E. The child needs to be quiet and physically in control by the end of the time-out or it is extended.

386.

Which of the following is true about brain growth during infancy and young children?

A. Enormous growth only occurs in the branching (the number is fixed) of dendrites, and the multiplication of complex synaptic junctions occurs.
B. Growth only occurs in the multiplication of complex synaptic junctions.
C. Enormous growth in the number and branching of dendrites, and the multiplication of complex synaptic junctions occurs.
D. Growth occurs in the number and branching of the dendrites, while the complex synaptic junctions do not develop further.
E. The human brain doubles in size postnatally.

387.

Which of the following is the <u>most</u> important factor in determining adaptive behavior for children raised in institutions?

A. Nutrition
B. Cleanliness
C. Sunlight
D. Amount of enrichment in adult-infant social interactions
E. Enrichment that occurs between the ages of 3 and 6 years of age, when children are more cognitive

388.

Which of the following cognitive stages of development might be seen in a 4-year-old child with acute leukemia during her therapy?

A. Magical thinking
B. Concrete operations
C. Formal operations
D. Peer acceptance is a concern
E. Do not perceive their illness as punishment for misdeeds

389.

All of the following are true regarding the treatment of chronic illnesses in children between the ages of 2 and 7 years of age <u>except</u>:

A. The <u>most</u> importment thing is to minimize separation from parents.
B. It is better to explain concrete aspects of procedures—the room for the surgery, the masks worn by the staff, etc.—rather than the procedure itself.
C. Pain is overdiagnosed and overtreated in hospitalized children.
D. The child should be allowed choices in the medical routine.
E. At these ages it helps to utilize the child life staff.

390.

A 7-year-old boy is brought to the office by his father for an annual checkup. During the course of the evaluation, his father complains that his son and his 5-year-old sister are always fighting. He says that his son hits his sister and nothing he can do prevents them from fighting. The boy is an "A" student and has no behavior problems in school. The past medical history and physical examination are completely normal.

Which of the following are appropriate coping skills for parents to deal with sibling rivalry?

A. Take sides.
B. Allow children to vent negative feelings.
C. It is appropriate to serve as a referee.
D. Use derogatory names.
E. Permit verbal but not physical abuse between siblings.

391.

Jane School is a 5-year-old girl who is brought to the office for a physical examination for kindergarten. Jane has been well and has been seen in the clinic only for an occasional cold and 2 episodes of otitis media when she was a year old. Her mother expresses concern that Jane is "painfully shy." She has never participated in a daycare program, and she spends most of her time at home with her mother.

Jane has reached all of her developmental milestones at appropriate ages, currently speaks very well in sentences, is able to dress herself without assistance, and can balance on one foot without difficulty.

Her physical examination is entirely normal. However, numerous times during the visit, she is "corrected" by her mother—"sit up straight," "stop fidgeting," "act your age," "silly."

Which of the following might be helpful to Jane to become less shy?

A. Allow the mother to expect perfection but to know that it may not always occur.
B. Suggest that the child may need to feel "overly protected" sometimes.
C. It is best to focus on the child's mistakes so she won't make the same mistakes again.
D. Encourage her mother to not use "don't" and "no" phrases.
E. "Labels" can be very helpful, like "good" and "bad."

392.

A 5-year-old boy is brought into the office by his father, who complains that his son has been frightened of sleeping alone since the occurrence of a tornado near their home. The house did not sustain any damage, but the entire family was awakened by the "freight train" noise. The father notes that his son appears to be more timid now. As nighttime approaches, he becomes particularly fearful. He will not stay in his bed, and he is comforted only by sleeping with his parents. Additionally, he started having bed-wetting episodes since the tornado. The physical examination is normal, except you note that the child is very "clingy and whiny."

Which of the following choices is warranted?

    A. Laboratory tests are usually required in this situation to help rule out organic etiologies for the bed-wetting.
    B. Children should not be empowered to conquer their fears.
    C. His fears should be validated; and to combat his fear of separation by a natural disaster, the parents should reassure him that they will all be together.
    D. Findings on physical examination in this situation are usually abnormal.
    E. They should watch television shows with tornadoes to help alleviate his anxiety.

HEALTH SUPERVISION

393.

During a scheduled well-child visit, a 6-month-old girl is noted to be pale on physical examination. Her hemoglobin is 8.9 g/dL. She is exclusively breastfed. Her mother follows a strict vegan diet.

Which of the following findings is most likely to be identified upon examination of a peripheral smear from this 6-month-old girl?

A. Microcytosis
B. Macrocytosis
C. Thrombocytopenia
D. Atypical lymphocytes
E. Burr and helmet cells

394.

A 20-month-old boy is rushed to the emergency room because, according to his parents, he "turned blue after hitting his head on a chair." Although he did not cry after hitting his head, his parents are also concerned that he seriously injured himself because he "jerked his arms and legs while on the floor." His parents go on to state that their son "started breathing again less than a minute" after he fell. On physical exam, his vital signs are stable. He is alert and willingly plays with a toy while sitting on his mother's lap. There is a 1 cm x 2 cm hematoma on his left forehead. No associated bony abnormalities are noted. Neurological examination is appropriate for his age.

Which of the following is the next best step in the treatment of this child?

A. CT scan of the head.
B. Examination of the fundi following dilation of the pupils.
C. Plain radiographs of the facial bones.
D. EEG.
E. Reassure the parents that no further workup is necessary.

395.

A 2-year-old African-American boy with sickle-cell disease presents for a scheduled well-child examination. His only daily medication is oral penicillin prophylaxis. He has been hospitalized twice for evaluation of "rule-out-sepsis fever." Review of his immunization record indicates that he has received all appropriate vaccinations, including *Haemophilus influenzae* type b (Hib) and heptavalent pneumococcal conjugate vaccine (PCV-7).

Which of the following represents the most appropriate recommendation in regard to the need for administering additional vaccines during this visit?

A. He does not require any vaccinations.
B. He should receive both an additional Hib and PCV7 vaccine.
C. He should receive both a PCV-7 vaccine and a 23 valent pneumococcal polysaccharide vaccine (PPV23).
D. He should receive a PPV-23 vaccine.
E. He should receive a Hib vaccine.

396.

The parents of a 3-year-old boy request that their son receive the "nasal flu vaccine" because he is afraid of getting a shot.

Which of the following statements represents a contraindication to the administration of the live attenuated influenza vaccine?

A. The patient takes daily salicylate therapy due to coronary artery abnormalities following Kawasaki disease diagnosed 6 months earlier.
B. The patient has been diagnosed with autism.
C. The patient takes daily antimicrobial therapy for prophylaxis against urinary tract infection associated with vesicoureteral reflux.
D. The patient takes daily valproic acid therapy for control of a seizure disorder.
E. The patient has a prior history of surgery to correct a deviated nasal septum.

397.

Following a normal examination during a scheduled well-child visit, a 15-month-old boy is scheduled to receive MMR and varicella vaccines. His mother, a recent immigrant from Central America, is currently pregnant with twins at 26-weeks gestation. During her first pregnancy, she received no prenatal care. Routine prenatal labs during her current pregnancy indicate that she is rubella non-immune and varicella immune.

Which of the following recommendations is most appropriate in this patient?

A. Both MMR and varicella vaccines should be delayed until after delivery of the twins.
B. Administer varicella vaccine during this visit and delay MMR vaccine until after delivery of the twins.
C. Administer varicella and MMR vaccines one week after the mother receives immune globulin.
D. Administer both varicella and MMR vaccines at this visit.
E. Administer varicella and monovalent rubeola vaccine at this visit.

398.

A 3-year-old boy, recently adopted from Honduras, is diagnosed with varicella. His adoptive mother provides daily care to several neighborhood children in her home while their parents are at work.

Which of the following choices describes the most appropriate intervention in those children exposed to the index case?

A. All unimmunized contacts of the index case with no prior history of natural varicella infection should receive chemoprophylaxis with oral acyclovir for 10 days.
B. Both immunized and non-immunized contacts with no prior history of natural varicella infection should receive chemoprophylaxis with oral acyclovir for 10 days.
C. Within 48 hours, all unimmunized contacts with no prior history of natural varicella infection should receive varicella vaccine and begin chemoprophylaxis with oral acyclovir for 14 days.
D. All unimmunized contacts ≥ 12 months with no prior history of natural varicella infection should receive varicella vaccine within 72 hours of exposure.
E. Varicella vaccine should be administered to all contacts of the index case ≤ 12 months of age.

399.

An 8-year-old child with sickle-cell disease presents for a well-child examination prior to returning to school.

Which of the following would indicate that this patient has met current recommendations for the use of pneumococcal vaccine(s) in patients with sickle-cell disease and other hemoglobinopathies?

   A. Heptavalent pneumococcal conjugate vaccine (PCV7) at 2, 4, 6, and 12 months of age
   B. Twenty-three (23) valent pneumococcal polysaccharide vaccine (PPV23) at 2, 4, 6, and 12 months of age
   C. PCV7 at 2, 4, and 6 months of age; PPV23 at 12 and 24 months of age
   D. PCV7 at 2, 4, 6, 12, and 24 months of age; PPV23 at 5 years of age
   E. PCV7 at 2, 4, 6, and 12 months of age; PPV23 at 2 and 5 years of age

400.

The parents of a 7-year-old boy born at 27-weeks gestation present with concerns about their son's behavior both at home and at school. Although his current signs and symptoms, along with information provided by his parents and teacher, are highly suggestive of attention deficit hyperactivity disorder (ADHD), his parents are concerned that he should not take stimulant medication because of "all of his other medical problems."

Which of the following conditions would preclude a trial of stimulant medication in this patient?

   A. Structural heart defect
   B. Seizure disorder
   C. Short gut syndrome
   D. Motor tics
   E. Hydronephrosis associated with renal insufficiency

401.

During a health maintenance visit, the parents of a 7-year-old boy request that he receive the "nasal flu vaccine" rather than the "flu shot."

Which of the following represents a contraindication to use of the live attenuated influenza virus vaccine?

   A. A history of migraine headaches associated with an aura
   B. A history of a seizure disorder
   C. A household contact requiring daily corticosteroid therapy
   D. A history of reactive airways disease
   E. Vaccination in a previous year(s) with the killed influenza virus vaccine

402.

A 17-month-old boy presents for a routine health maintenance visit. Review of his immunization records indicates that he should receive a MMR vaccination.

Which of the following is a contraindication to administering this vaccine?

  A. Administration of immune globulin 2 months earlier for treatment of immune thrombocytopenic purpura
  B. Daily therapy with inhaled steroids for control of asthma
  C. History of an anaphylactic reaction to baker's yeast
  D. Household member with HIV/AIDS
  E. Daily therapy with valproic acid for control of a seizure disorder

403.

A 6-month-old boy presents for a routine health maintenance visit. Review of his immunization records indicates that he should receive a DTaP vaccination.

Which of the following is a contraindication to administering this vaccine?

  A. Temperature of > 39.5° C (103.1° F) within 24 hours of administration of a previous dose of a DTaP vaccine
  B. Family history of sudden infant death syndrome
  C. Seizure within one week of administration of a previous dose of a DTaP vaccine
  D. A seizure disorder consistent with infantile spasms
  E. Encephalopathy within one month of administration of a previous dose of a DTaP vaccine

404.

Shortly after returning to the United States following a trip to Europe, a 14-month-old boy is confirmed by laboratory testing to have measles. During the week prior to his diagnosis, the patient attended a day care center while his parents worked.

Which of the following outlines the appropriate recommendation for prevention of spread of disease through vaccination of infants ≤ 11 months of age attending the same day care center as this patient?

  A. Administer any live measles-containing vaccine to all infants 1–11 months of age.
  B. Administer any live measles-containing vaccine to all infants 1–5 months of age.
  C. Administer only the monovalent form of measles vaccine to all infants 1–11 months of age.
  D. Administer any live measles-containing vaccine to all infants 6–11 months of age.
  E. No intervention is indicated due to the presence of passively acquired maternal measles antibodies in this age group.

405.

You meet baby girl Johnson in the newborn nursery. You have taken care of Mrs. Johnson's other two children and from discussions you had with the mother, you knew to expect this new child. The mother had an unremarkable pregnancy, labor, and vaginal delivery and had routine medical care starting the second month of her pregnancy. The infant was a healthy-appearing newborn that had been given APGAR scores of 9 at one minute and 9 at five minutes. Her physical examination was entirely normal and she was breastfeeding well. You relate this information to the mother and during the conversation, she states that she knows you will want to see this infant in one week for a health supervision visit but has forgotten when the next visit should be.

When should the second post-natal health supervision visit be?

A. No routine scheduled visits are necessary because this is her 3rd child
B. 1 month
C. 2 weeks
D. 2 months
E. 6 weeks

406.

Which of the following vaccines are usually given as subcutaneous injections?

A. MMR, IPV, varicella
B. MMR, DTaP, varicella
C. MMR, DTaP
D. MMR, DTaP, IPV
E. DTaP, IPV, varicella

407.

You are about to immunize a 13-month-old girl with MMR and varicella vaccines. You are called to an emergency C-Section and your immunization nurse accompanies you. Just before the two of you are called away, she had already prepared the MMR and varicella vaccines and placed them into their syringes for administration. She returns to the office after 1 hour.

Which of the following is true?

A. She may administer both.
B. She may administer the varicella vaccine but not the MMR vaccine.
C. She may administer the MMR vaccine but not the varicella vaccine.
D. She may administer neither.
E. She may administer the MMR now and she may administer the varicella vaccine if the color of the material has not turned light pink.

408.

A 16-year-old teenager presents for his first hepatitis B immunization. He otherwise is healthy and is a member of the weightlifting and football teams. While the nurse is administering his vaccine, he says he is dizzy and then drops to the floor.

Which of the following is the likely etiology of this episode?

A. Anaphylaxis to the protein portion of the vaccine
B. Hypoglycemia
C. Anabolic steroid interaction with the vaccine
D. Idiosyncratic reaction to mercury in the vaccine
E. Syncope

409.

Which of the following are the generally preferred sites for most intramuscular vaccines?

A. Anterolateral aspect of the upper thigh and the deltoid region of the upper arm
B. Anterolateral aspect of the upper thigh and the volar region of the lower arm
C. Anteromedial aspect of the upper thigh, the upper outer aspect of the buttocks, and the deltoid region of the upper arm
D. Anteromedial aspect of the upper thigh and the volar region of the lower arm
E. Anywhere you can get the squirmy kid

410.

Needles for IM vaccination should be long enough to reach adequate muscle tissue.

Which of the following needle sizes are appropriate for each age group?

A. 1" for 4-month-old infant for thigh penetration; 1" for 130-kg male for deltoid penetration
B. 2" for 4-month-old infant for thigh penetration; 2" for 130-kg male for deltoid penetration
C. 1/2" for 4-month-old infant for thigh penetration; 1" for 130-kg male for deltoid penetration
D. 1" for 4-month-old infant for thigh penetration; 2" for 130-kg male for deltoid penetration
E. 1/2" for 4-month-old infant for thigh penetration; 2" for 130-kg male for deltoid penetration

411.

Sally is a 2-month-old infant who presents for routine immunization. She is healthy and does not have any known contraindications to current vaccine products. She received hepatitis B vaccination in the newborn nursery before discharge.

Which of the following vaccines should she receive today?

A. Hepatitis B, DTaP, Hib, rotavirus, pneumococcal only
B. Hepatitis B, DTaP, Hib, rotavirus, IPV, pneumococcal
C. Hepatitis B, DTaP, rotavirus, pneumococcal only
D. DTaP, Hib, IPV, rotavirus, pneumococcal only
E. DTaP, Hib, IPV, MMR, rotavirus, pneumococcal

412.

A 14-year-old girl presents for routine checkup for camp physical. In reviewing her immunization records, you note that she has not received the varicella vaccine.

Which of the following is correct?

A. If she has not had a history of varicella, she should receive one dose of vaccine today; no further doses are required.
B. Regardless of her varicella history, she should receive the varicella vaccine.
C. Since she is older than 12, it is best not to give the vaccine now.
D. If she has not had a history of varicella, she should receive 2 doses of vaccine at least 4 weeks apart.
E. If a varicella titer is sent and is positive, she still may be at risk and thus she should receive vaccine.

413.

A 5-year-old girl has not received any of her immunizations. Her birth mother was schizophrenic and never took the child in for well-child checkups. The child now lives with her grandparents, and her mother is receiving needed psychiatric treatment. On physical examination, she appears to be in good health and developmentally is appropriate for age.

Which of the following vaccines should she receive today?

A. DTaP, hepatitis B, MMR, varicella, IPV, hepatitis A
B. DTaP, hepatitis B, MMR, varicella, IPV, Hib, hepatitis A
C. Td, hepatitis B, MMR, varicella, IPV, hepatitis A
D. Td, hepatitis B, MMR, varicella, IPV, Hib, hepatitis A
E. Td, MMR, varicella, IPV, hepatitis A

414.

A 5-year-old child received her first set of vaccines today. She is "way behind" in her immunizations.

Which of the following is the earliest (and recommended) time for her to return for her next set of immunizations?

A. 6 weeks
B. 2 months
C. 4 weeks
D. 2 weeks
E. 7 weeks

415.

A 5-year-old child received her first set of vaccines today. She is "way behind" in her immunizations. Today she received the following vaccines: DTaP, HBV, MMR, varicella, IPV, and hepatitis A.

When she returns in 4 weeks for her next set of immunizations, what should she receive?

A. DTaP, HBV, MMR, varicella, IPV, hepatitis A
B. DTaP, HBV, MMR, IPV
C. Tdap, HBV, IPV, hepatitis A
D. Td, HBV, MMR, IPV
E. DTaP, varicella, hepatitis A

416.

A 10-year-old boy has not received any immunizations. He is currently healthy. He had varicella at the age of 3 documented by a physician visit.

Which of the following immunizations should he receive today?

A. Hepatitis B, MMR, Tdap, IPV, hepatitis A, HPV
B. Hepatitis B, MMR, Tdap, IPV, Hib, hepatitis A
C. Hepatitis B, MMR, DTaP, IPV, Hib, hepatitis A
D. Hepatitis B, MMR, DTaP, IPV, hepatitis A, HPV
E. Hepatitis B, MMR, Td, IPV, Hib, varicella, hepatitis A, HPV

417.

An 11-year-old girl received her first set of immunizations today. She is "way behind."

Which of the following is the recommended time for her to return for her next set of immunizations?

A. 2 weeks
B. 12 weeks
C. 4 weeks
D. 6 weeks
E. 8 weeks

418.

A mother brings in her 2-month-old for immunizations. The mother is concerned about the number of vaccines the baby will receive and asks if there are any problems with simultaneous vaccinations.

Because of decreased immunogenicity, which of the following vaccine pairs is it best <u>not</u> to give at the same visit?

A. DTaP and IPV
B. DTaP and MMR
C. MMR and IPV
D. MMR and hepatitis B
E. None; all of the vaccine pairs can be given at the same visit without significantly diminishing immunogenicity

419.

A 10-month-old who received her first set of immunizations (hepatitis B, IPV, DTaP, Hib, rotavirus, pneumococcal) at the age of 2 months has been lost to follow-up until today.

Because 8 months have intervened since her last vaccination, which vaccine(s) should she "start over from scratch" and assume that she has no immunity?

A. None; she does not require reinstitution of the entire series for any of these vaccines
B. Hepatitis B
C. IPV
D. Hepatitis B, IPV, DTaP, Hib
E. Hepatitis B, DTaP

420.

A 10-year-old girl presents for routine evaluation. She lived in Louisiana until 3 years ago and has lived in multiple cities over the last few years because her father is a truck driver. She is about to enroll in your local school district. Documentation of her immunization status cannot be found, and the courthouse in Louisiana that held her records has been destroyed by a hurricane. Her father cannot reliably tell you which immunizations she received or when. She has never had chicken pox.

Which of the following is the best plan?

A. Reinstitute the entire immunization sequence for hepatitis B, hepatitis A, polio, measles, mumps, rubella, varicella, and tetanus (1 Tdap followed by Td at usual intervals; 1 Tdap is appropriate for pertussis).

B. Reinstitute the entire immunization sequence for hepatitis B, polio, measles, mumps, rubella, diphtheria, pneumonococcus, and tetanus (1 Tdap followed by Td at usual intervals; 1 Tdap is appropriate for pertussis).

C. Reinstitute the entire immunization sequence for hepatitis B, polio, measles, mumps, rubella, *Haemophilus influenzae*, pertussis, diphtheria, and tetanus.

D. Since she is 10, and assuming she had some vaccines as a child, only give her Tdap, hepatitis A, and Hepatitis B now.

E. Send titers and see if she is immune.

421.

A 5-year-old child presents with a fever of 102° F and earache. She is quite talkative and feels better after acetaminophen. You diagnose her with a left otitis media. You note that she is due for an MMR, IPV, and DTaP today.

Which of the following do you recommend?

A. Have her return in 10 days for the vaccines.
B. Administer only the IPV today; return for the MMR and DTaP in 2 weeks.
C. Have her return for check-up in 3 days; if afebrile then immunize her.
D. Administer the MMR, IPV, and DTaP today.
E. Observe her in the office for 2 more hours; if she is still afebrile, then administer the vaccines.

HEMATOLOGY / ONCOLOGY

422.

Which of the following is the <u>least</u> common finding in a new pediatric leukemia patient?

A. Bone pain
B. Fevers
C. Hepatosplenomegaly
D. Platelets < 50,000
E. WBC > 100,000

423.

A 13-year-old volleyball player complains of pain after trauma. Her x-ray is below:

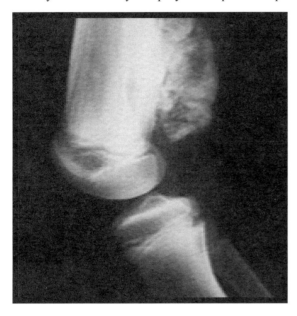

Which of the following is the most likely diagnosis?

A. Ewing's sarcoma
B. Osteosarcoma
C. Histiocytosis
D. Osteomyelitis
E. Bone lymphoma

424.

Which of the following are indications for red blood cell transfusion in a sickle-cell anemia patient with acute chest syndrome?

A. Pneumonia, TIA (transient ischemic attack), Hg < 7 g/dL
B. Pneumonia, TIA, Hg < 7 g/dL, pain crisis
C. Pneumonia, TIA, surgery
D. Hg < 7 g/dL, surgery
E. Pneumonia, TIA, Hg < 7 g/dL, pain crisis, surgery

425.

Which of the following is the most dangerous? (ANC = absolute neutrophil count).

A. ANC = 100 that is virus-induced
B. ANC = 500 that is chemotherapy-induced
C. ANC = 0 that is due to autoimmune neutropenia
D. ANC = 100 that is due to Kostmann syndrome
E. ANC = 50 that is due to cyclic neutropenia

426.

A 10-year-old presents with morning headaches, emesis, precocious puberty, bitemporal hemianopsia, and progressive behavior changes.

Which of the following is the most likely diagnosis?

A. Retinoblastoma
B. CNS germ cell tumor
C. Glioblastoma multiforme
D. CNS leukemia
E. Histiocytosis

427.

A mother felt a mass in the abdomen of her otherwise healthy 5-year-old son. The CT is shown below.

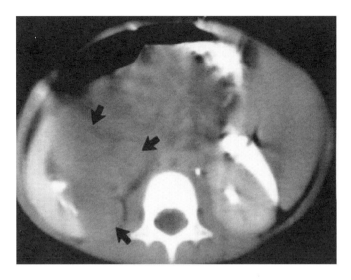

Which of the following is the most likely diagnosis?

A. Wilms tumor
B. Hepatoblastoma
C. Burkitt lymphoma
D. Hepatocellular carcinoma
E. Neuroblastoma

428.

A 17-year-old African-American female with patellar dislocation develops leg swelling and tenderness on the 3rd post-operative day. The aPPT is prolonged to 46 sec (23–33), and there is no correction of the aPTT in 1:1 mix with normal plasma.

Which of the following would be the next most helpful test to order?

A. Low protein C
B. Elevated homocysteine
C. Prothrombin gene mutation
D. Factor V Leiden
E. Lupus anticoagulant

429.

Pre-operative assessment of a 16-year-old boy prior to open reduction of a traumatic fracture of the humerus reveals frequent epistaxis. His mother has menorrhagia. The aPTT is 38 seconds (23–33 sec); the bleeding time is 12.5 minutes (3.5–9.5 min).

Which of the following is the best test to order now?

A. Ristocetin co-factor activity
B. von Willebrand multimers
C. von Willebrand antigen
D. Factor VIII level
E. Platelet count

430.

Which of the following is a reason to give trimethoprim/sulfamethoxazole to cancer patients?

A. *Pneumocystis jiroveci* (formerly *P. carinii*) prophylaxis
B. Decrease febrile neutropenia
C. UTI prophylaxis
D. Central line prophylaxis
E. To enhance efficacy of methotrexate

431.

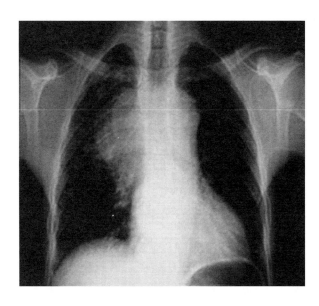

Which of the following best describes the "B" symptoms associated with the disease seen in this chest x-ray?

A. Weight loss > 10%, night sweats, bone pain
B. Weight loss > 10%, night sweats, fevers
C. Weight loss > 10%, night sweats, bone pain, and rash
D. Night sweats and bone pain
E. All of the answers are correct.

432.

Which of the following is the most likely diagnosis in this infant who presents with severe constipation and an extremely elevated alpha-fetoprotein (AFP)?

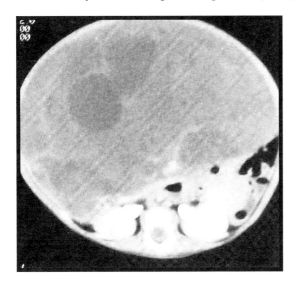

A. Neuroblastoma
B. Hepatoblastoma
C. Burkitt lymphoma
D. Wilms tumor
E. Germ cell tumor

433.

Which of the following tumors/cancers are associated with NF-2 (neurofibromatosis Type 2)?

A. Leukemia, malignant peripheral nerve sheath tumors (MPNST), and ependymoma
B. Leukemia, malignant peripheral nerve sheath tumors (MPNST), and malignant gliomas
C. Acoustic neuroma and malignant gliomas
D. Acoustic neuroma and ependymoma
E. All of the answers are correct.

434.

Which of the following is the appropriate test/treatment for a child with 3 weeks of back pain and tingling in her hands?

A. Emergency MRI of the spine
B. Cervical/thoracic spine x-rays
C. CT chest and spine
D. CBC with smear
E. Trial of NSAIDs

435.

Which of the following are associated with Coombs-negative (direct antibody test negative) causes of neonatal jaundice?

A. α thalassemia
B. α thalassemia, G6PD deficiency, hereditary spherocytosis (HS)
C. α thalassemia, β thalassemia, G6PD deficiency, hereditary spherocytosis (HS)
D. ABO or minor group incompatibilities, α thalassemia, β thalassemia, G6PD deficiency, hereditary spherocytosis (HS)
E. ABO or minor group incompatibilities, α thalassemia, β thalassemia, G6PD deficiency, hereditary spherocytosis (HS), sickle cell anemia

436.

A hemoglobin electrophoresis and lab is presented for a 3-year-old patient with microcytic anemia:

Hemoglobin A = 30%   Normal > 90%
Hemoglobin S = 60 %   Normal 0%
Hemoglobin F = 15%   Normal < 2%
Hemoglobin A_2 = 5 %   Normal 2–3.5%
Hemoglobin = 10.0 g/dL,
Hematocrit = 31%,
MCV = 60

Which of the following is the correct interpretation?

A. Sickle trait
B. Homozygous sickle-cell anemia
C. Homozygous sickle-cell anemia on hydroxyurea
D. Sickle β thalassemia
E. Homozygous sickle-cell anemia after transfusion of pRBCs

437.

Which of the following is the most common reason for thrombocytopenia in a child?

A. Artifact "clumping"
B. Viral or drug-induced
C. ITP (autoimmune thrombocytopenia purpura)
D. Leukemia
E. TTP

438.

For which of the following does an abnormally prolonged aPTT correct with 1:1 mixing study?

A. Lupus anticoagulant
B. Heparin effect
C. FXI deficiency
D. FVII deficiency
E. Heparin effect or FXI deficiency

439.

All the clotting factors are made in the liver, except which of the following?

A. Fibrinogen (I)
B. Prothrombin (II)
C. FV
D. FVII
E. FVIII

440.

Which of the following clotting factors are depleted with warfarin therapy?

A. Prothrombin (II), FV, FVII, FVIII
B. Prothrombin (II), FV, FVII, FX
C. Prothrombin (II), FV, FVII, FX, Protein C, Protein S
D. Prothrombin (II), FVII, FIX, FX
E. Prothrombin (II), FVII, FIX, FX, Protein C, Protein S

441.

Which of the following is seen first in acute liver failure?

A. Prolonged PT
B. Prolonged aPTT
C. Prolonged thrombin time
D. Prolonged PT and prolonged aPTT
E. All of the answers are correct.

442.

Which of the following is primarily a neutrophil problem?

A. Hyper IgE syndrome
B. Hyper IgM syndrome
C. Bruton agammaglobulinemia
D. Bloom syndrome
E. DiGeorge syndrome

443.

Which is likely to be most mild: alpha-thalassemia major, beta-thalassemia major, or both diseases concurrently and in what part of the world are both diseases seen frequently?

A. Beta-thalassemia, both are seen in the Mediterranean
B. Both alpha-thalassemia and beta-thalassemia, both are seen in the Mediterranean
C. Alpha-thalassemia, both are seen in Asia
D. Beta-thalassemia, both are seen in Africa
E. Concurrent alpha-thalassemia and beta-thalassemia, both are seen in Africa

444.

Which of the following is activated protein C resistance (APC resistance) associated with?

A. Elevated homocysteine
B. Factor V Leiden mutation
C. Prothrombin gene mutation
D. MTHFR (methylenetetrahydrofolate reductase) mutation
E. Increase survival in sepsis

445.

Three weeks after a varicella infection, a 4-year-old African-American boy presents with a normal physical exam except for petechiae and bruising. His labs show: Hg = 12.1 g/dL, blood type A+, WBC = 6.3, ANC = 800, Platelets = 3,000.

Which of the following would be most appropriate to do next?

A. Give anti-D immunoglobin
B. Start prednisone
C. Transfuse one unit of phoresed platelets
D. Arrange for a bone marrow aspirate
E. Send ANA

446.

Which of the following statements about long-term side effects of cancer treatment is/are true?

A. Cardiomyopathy can occur from doxorubicin up to 10 years later; etoposide can give a secondary leukemia in the first 3 years; and methotrexate is known to cause infertility, especially in males.

B. Cardiomyopathy can occur from doxorubicin up to 10 years later; etoposide can give a secondary leukemia in the first 3 years; and breast cancer is increased in survivors of Hodgkin disease.

C. Cardiomyopathy can occur from doxorubicin up to 10 years later; etoposide can give a secondary leukemia in the first 3 years; and pulmonary fibrosis is a known long-term side effect of vincristine.

D. Etoposide can give a secondary leukemia in the first 3 years; methotrexate is known to cause infertility, especially in males; and breast cancer is increased in survivors of Hodgkin disease.

E. All of the answers are correct.

447.

A 3-year-old boy has chronic diarrhea, failure to thrive, recurrent infections, eczema, and platelets = 56,000. IgA is elevated and IgM is low.

Which of the following is the most likely diagnosis?

A. TAR (thrombocytopenia absent radii)
B. Fanconi anemia
C. Wiskott-Aldrich syndrome
D. Shwachman-Diamond syndrome (SDS)
E. HUS (hemolytic uremic syndrome)

448.

Here is an MRI of a child's brain tumor.

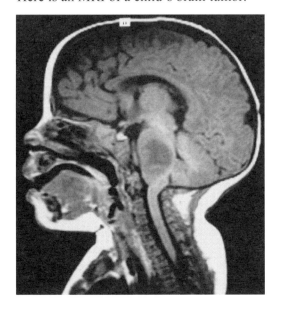

Which of the following is the type of brain tumor and its likely survival rate?

A. Ependymoma 50%
B. Brain stem glioma 40%
C. Medulloblastoma 85%
D. Brain stem glioma < 5%
E. Medulloblastoma 30%

449.

A 7-year-old girl with a history of sickle-cell disease presents to the emergency room with her parents, who are concerned that she can "no longer even go up stairs without getting short of breath." Her parents deny associated symptoms but do relate that their older daughter was "sent home from school with a rash" several days earlier. Laboratory tests include hemoglobin of 5.1g/dL and a reticulocyte count: 0.1%.

Which of the following best describes the likely appearance of the rash in this patient's sister?

A. A fine macular papular "sandpaper-like" rash on the trunk
B. Multiple, elevated, slightly warm and pruritic oval shaped plaques on the trunk and extremities
C. Multiple slightly raised scaling plaque-like oval lesions on the posterior trunk and upper portions of the anterior trunk
D. Multiple widespread pruritic clear vesicles on an erythematous base
E. Distinct erythema of the cheeks associated with a macular "lacy" appearing rash on the upper extremities

450.

The parents of a 3-year-old Caucasian female present with concerns that their daughter tires easily, will frequently complain of a "stomachache, and is not interested in playing. On physical exam she is afebrile but appears lethargic. Blood pressure is 75/50 and heart rate is 140 beats/minute. Her sclera are noted to be icteric, and her spleen is enlarged. Laboratory findings include hemoglobin of 8.2g/dL and an indirect bilirubin of 6.8mg/dL. An abdominal ultrasound is positive for several gallstones and moderate enlargement of the spleen.

Which of the following additional laboratory studies is most likely to be present upon further evaluation of this patient?

A. Spherocytes on a peripheral smear
B. Elevated serum ammonia level
C. Elevated serum lead level
D. A positive indirect Coombs
E. Elevated levels of serum amylase and lipase

451.

An 18-month-old boy is admitted for dehydration associated with fever and refusal to eat. He has had two previous hospitalizations for cellulitis and dehydration and a third for pneumonia. On physical examination he is estimated to be 5% dehydrated. His temperature is 103.2° F. He appears ill but with no evidence of associated meningeal signs. His exam is positive for stomatitis, oral ulcerations and cervical lymphadenopathy. A complete blood count (CBC) reveals an absolute neutrophil count (ANC) of 406 cells per mm^3 with no other associated abnormalities.

Which of the following findings is most likely to be identified upon further evaluation of this patient?

A. A positive blood culture for *Clostridium perfringens*
B. Elevated liver function tests
C. A positive Western blot for HIV
D. An absent thymus on chest x-ray
E. A bone marrow aspirate consistent with acute lymphoblastic leukemia

---

452.

A 6-year-old boy with a history of developmental delay and hearing loss presents for additional evaluation. His teacher reports that both his cognitive and language skills are significantly behind those of his peers. Both his teacher and his mother also report that he is irritable and will frequently complain of stomach pain. During laboratory evaluation a peripheral smear reveals the presence of blue granules of various sizes dispersed throughout the cytoplasm of the red blood cells.

Which of the following laboratory findings is most likely to also be identified upon further evaluation of this patient?

A. Elevated levels of serum amylase and lipase
B. Decreased levels of serum ceruloplasmin
C. Decreased levels of serum alpha-1 antitrypsin
D. Decreased levels of blood zinc protoporphyrin (ZPP)
E. Elevated levels of blood erythrocyte protoporphyrin (EP)

453.

A 3-year-old boy presents for a follow-up visit to re-evaluate his growth parameters. His past medical history is positive for poor weight gain, irritability, and frequent episodes of diarrhea, originally thought to be due to a milk protein allergy. On physical exam he has prominent periorbital ecchymoses. His abdomen is distended and associated with a nodular mass in the right flank.

Which of the following findings is most likely to be identified upon further evaluation?

A. A non-calcified abdominal mass on CT extending into the renal veins
B. Hydronephrosis on renal ultrasound
C. Renal enlargement associated with several cysts on renal ultrasound
D. An abdominal mass associated with "stippled calcifications" on CT
E. Posterior urethral valves and severe vesicoureteric reflux

INFECTIOUS DISEASES

454.

A 16-year-old girl presents with left ankle arthritis and a pustular lesion on her right toe and left hand. She is sexually active and reports that she began her menses today. The skin overlying her arthritis is exquisitely tender.

Which of the following would be the best treatment?

A. Ciprofloxacin
B. Cefazolin
C. Ceftriaxone
D. Ampicillin
E. Doxycycline

455.

Which of the following would be an indication for hospitalization for pelvic inflammatory disease (PID)?

A. Confirmed diagnosis of PID.
B. Had one episode of nausea earlier in the day.
C. Urine pregnancy test is positive.
D. No improvement after 4 hours of oral therapy.
E. Appendicitis has been excluded as an etiology.

456.

A 17-year-old male returns from a spring break holiday in the Caribbean. After 5 days he notes a small tender papule with surrounding erythema on the shaft of his penis. It evolves over several days into a pustule and now has become painful with tender lymphadenopathy in his groin area. You note an exudate in the ulcer base and you get a Gram stain, which shows the following:

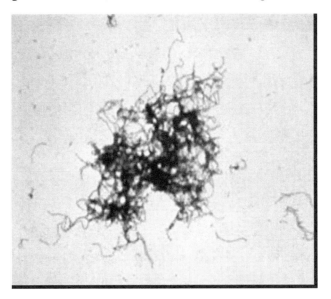

Which of the following is the most likely organism responsible?

A. *Treponema pallidum*
B. *Chlamydia trachomatis*
C. *Chlamydia pneumoniae*
D. *Haemophilus ducreyi*
E. *Klebsiella granulomatis*

457.

A 14-year-old girl presents with complaints of vaginal itching. You do an exam and discuss with her "safe sex" and age-appropriate anticipatory guidance. During the interview, she begins to cry and says that she has been sexually active with a boy on several occasions. She is worried because he is older and is "more experienced" than her. On further questioning, she thinks he might have syphilis. On further exam, you note that she has a chancre on her vulvar area.

Besides testing for other STDs, which of the following is the recommended treatment for her?

A. Penicillin V-K 250 mg PO qid x 10 days
B. Pen G benzathine 2.4 million units IM x 1 dose
C. Pen G benzathine 2.4 million units IM q week x 3 weeks
D. Doxycycline 100 mg PO bid x 4 weeks
E. Penicillin G 18 million units IV divided q 4–6 hours x 10 days

---

458.

In a child with otitis media, which of the following is <u>not</u> a risk factor for *Streptococcus pneumoniae* resistance?

A. Daycare attendance
B. Recent antibiotic usage
C. Age < 2 years
D. Concurrent viral infection
E. Recurrent otitis media

459.

A 5-year-old child presents with sore throat.

Which of the following findings would make *Streptococcus pyogenes* more likely?

A. Tender cervical lymphadenopathy
B. Cough
C. Rhinorrhea
D. Nasal congestion
E. Sneezing

460.

Which of the following is/are true about GABHS (group A beta-hemolytic streptococcal) infection?

A. Rheumatic fever occurs only from pharyngeal strains of GABHS.
B. Post-streptococcal glomerulonephritis can occur even with appropriate therapy.
C. Post-strep GN can occur from skin or pharyngeal strains.
D. Treatment of strep pharyngitis with penicillin prevents rheumatic fever.
E. All of the choices are correct.

461.

A 1-day-old with no history of prenatal care presents with fever and mottling. The mother delivered the infant at home.

Which of the following presentations would be most likely for group B streptococcus at this age?

A. Septicemia
B. Septic arthritis
C. Meningitis
D. Osteomyelitis
E. Cellulitis

462.

Which of the following organisms would you be worried about if the question referred to ingestion of "goat cheese" or "uncooked hotdogs"?

A. *Enterococcus*
B. *E. coli*
C. *Listeria*
D. Group B streptococcus
E. *Pseudomonas*

463.

A 16-year-old male comes in with a rash on his trunk. He is an African-American with light-colored, crusty lesions on his back and chest. They seem to become lighter when exposed to sunlight. You do a scraping of one of the lesions, and the results are presented here:

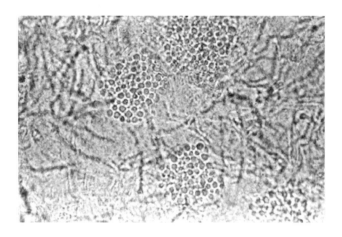

Which of the following is the diagnosis/organism responsible?

A. Tinea capitis
B. *Malassezia furfur* (*Pityrosporon orbiculare*)
C. *Candida albicans*
D. *Candida marneffei*
E. *Cryptococcus neoformans*

464.

A 13-year-old girl is due to receive her 2ⁿᵈ MMR. She also has a note from her school saying that she may have been exposed to a teacher with tuberculosis, and she requires PPD placement.

When is it appropriate to place her initial PPD if you give her MMR today?

A. Today
B. In 1 week
C. In 4 weeks
D. In 6 months
E. In 9 months

465.

A 12-year-old boy presents for evaluation. He lives in northwest Arkansas on a soybean and iguana farm. He has had 3 days of fever to 102° F. He has no lymphadenopathy but has a slight rash on his trunk. He likes to hunt with his brothers and has been in the rural woods of northern Arkansas every weekend for the past 9 years. He has removed numerous ticks from his body. His CBC shows a pancytopenia.

Which of the following is the most likely organism responsible?

A. *Ehrlichia*
B. *Klebsiella*
C. *Francisella*
D. *Legionella*
E. *Yersinia*

466.

Marla, a 4-year-old girl, steps on a dirty nail with cow feces on it. Her dog licks her foot after the injury. Her parents are rural migrant workers, and, as far as they know, she has not received any immunizations.

Which of the following tetanus immunizations/series should she receive today?

A. Td only
B. DTaP only
C. Td and tetanus IG
D. DTaP and tetanus IG
E. Wait 6 weeks to give her tetanus immunization. You must treat her with antibiotics first; otherwise, she may anaphylax to the vaccine, because she likely has natural tetanus antibodies.

467.

A 12-year-old girl presents with a draining lesion. Her mother reports she has had this lesion for 5–6 months, and it has not responded to cephalexin, doxycycline, or ciprofloxacin (um, given to her by a friend of the family, an internal medicine physician). She has no travel history. She spends the summers and winters at the local club indoor pool and remembers that she scraped her leg against the pool tile 6 months ago. Routine bacterial cultures have been negative except for methicillin-resistant *Staphylococcus epidermidis*, which was sensitive to ciprofloxacin.

Which of the following organisms is the most likely cause, based on her history?

A. *Francisella tularensis*
B. *Mycobacterium marinum*
C. *Mycobacterium tuberculosis*
D. *Mycobacterium pseudotuberculosis*
E. *Listeria monocytogenes*

468.

A 9-year-old girl is hospitalized with a history of intermittent daily fever of up to 103.3° F for the preceding 11 days. On the day prior to admission she developed a swollen, warm, and tender right ankle and left knee along with a non-pruritic erythematous macular rash associated with pale centers on the posterior trunk and extremities. During her hospitalization the rash is noted to be more prominent when she is febrile. An ECG shows evidence of a prolonged PR interval.

Which of the following results is most likely to be identified during additional evaluation of this patient?

A. Elevated antistreptolysin O (ASO) antibodies
B. Elevated antibody titers to *Rickettsia rickettsii*
C. Elevated antibody titers to Epstein Barr virus (EBV) early antigen
D. Positive screen for hepatitis B surface antigen (HBsAg)
E. Positive blood culture for *Salmonella typhi*

469.

A 14-year-old boy is transported to the emergency room following the rapid onset of altered mental status while waiting in the school nurse's office for his mother to pick him up from school. Upon arrival he is barely arousable and has a temperature of 104.2° F and blood pressure of 80/35. There is a purpuric and petechial rash covering his lower extremities and trunk. A Gram stain following scraping of a purpuric lesion reveals numerous Gram-negative diplococci. Further history reveals that the patient shares a bedroom with his twin brother.

Which of the following is the most appropriate treatment for the patient's brother?

A. Cefixime 400 mg PO twice daily for 2 days
B. Amoxicillin 1gram PO twice daily for 10 days
C. Doxycycline 100 mg PO twice daily for 10 days
D. Rifampin 600 mg PO twice daily for 2 days
E. Trimethoprim-sulfamethoxazole 160 mg/800 mg PO twice daily for 5 days

470.

An 18-year-old female presents to her college infirmary with a history of sudden onset of fever, myalgia, shortness of breath, vomiting, and rash. She is member of the soccer team and states that she had previously been well with the exception of a laceration on her left leg sustained 3 days earlier when she "fell and was cut by a cleat" on a teammate's shoe. On physical examination, her temperature is 104° F and blood pressure is 90/35. She is oriented but lethargic and has a diffuse, intensely erythematous rash most notable on her trunk and palms. Her tongue and conjunctiva are injected. The laceration itself appears inflamed with surrounding erythema and mucopurulent discharge. Laboratory results include an elevated white blood cell count and elevated hepatic and renal function tests.

Which of the following is the most likely cause of this patient's symptoms?

A. *Escherichia coli*
B. Epstein Barr virus
C. An extracellular toxin produced by *Staphylococcus aureus*
D. Hepatitis B virus
E. *Pseudomonas aeruginosa*

471.

The parents of an 11-year-old boy are called to their son's school because he "won't stop crying." Although he usually enjoys and does well in school, he started crying after his teacher commented how poor his writing had become over the last week. His parents also have noticed that his school work is uncharacteristically sloppy. On physical exam, his vital signs are stable; he is afebrile and continues to cry intermittently. When quieted by his parents, facial grimacing and facial tics are evident. On neurological exam, he is unable to perform finger-to-nose maneuvers or heal-to-toe walking. When asked to stand straight and hold out his hands, he struggles to remain still and often holds his hands in a pronated position.

During which one of the following diseases may individuals present with symptoms similar to this patient?

A. Acute rheumatic fever
B. Viral encephalitis
C. Lyme disease
D. Rocky mountain spotted fever
E. Infectious mononucleosis

472.

A 16-year-old male presents with a 5-day history of malaise, increased temperature, vague abdominal pain, and increasingly severe sore throat. On physical examination he appears moderately ill. His temperature is 103.2° F; other vital signs are appropriate for his age. His pharynx is erythematous; tonsils are somewhat enlarged with significant exudate. There is prominent cervical lymphadenopathy. The abdomen is slightly tender, and the spleen tip is palpable. A Monospot® test is positive, while a rapid strep antigen detection test is negative.

Which of the following most accurately describes the expected clinical outcome, results of laboratory testing, or most appropriate treatment plan in patients with infectious mononucleosis?

A. Acute symptoms usually resolve within 3–5 days if treatment with corticosteroids is initiated at the time of diagnosis.
B. The patient should receive a 10-day course of acyclovir to hasten recovery and prevent complications.
C. The patient should receive a 10-day course of antimicrobials to prevent complications from likely coinfection with group A streptococcus and/or *Mycoplasma pneumoniae.*
D. In the absence of splenomegaly, patients may return to contact sports 72 hours after becoming afebrile.
E. Younger patients with infectious mononucleosis are less likely to test positive for heterophile antibodies.

473.

After waiting in the office for 1 hour before being seen by a physician, a 14-month-old unimmunized infant who recently returned from an overseas trip is diagnosed with measles. Just yesterday he and his mother visited their neighbors who have twin boys aged 18 months. Both boys are scheduled for well-child examinations in 2 weeks, at which time they are to receive their first MMR vaccination.

Which of the following is the most appropriate next step in the treatment of the twin boys?

A. Administer MMR vaccine and immune globulin within 4 hours of exposure.
B. Administer MMR vaccine within 72 hours of exposure.
C. Administer immune globulin within 15 days of exposure.
D. Administer monovalent rubeola vaccine within 5 days of exposure.
E. Administer monovalent rubeola vaccine and immune globulin within 15 days of exposure.

474.

A 17-year-old male requires 15 sutures to repair a laceration obtained during football practice. Review of his immunization record shows that he received all recommended vaccines by the time of elementary school entry, with the last one recorded at age 5 years 4 months.

Which of the following scenarios would require that this patient receive a Tdap vaccination prior to discharge from the emergency room?

    A. He also received a Td vaccine at 14 years of age.
    B. He also received a Tdap vaccine at 10 years of age.
    C. He also received a Td vaccine at 10 years of age.
    D. He also received a Tdap vaccine at 12 years of age.
    E. He also received a Td vaccine at 10 and at 15 years of age.

475.

During a prenatal ultrasound at 24 weeks gestation, significant fetal edema is identified in the subcutaneous tissue, pleura, liver, and abdomen. There is also evidence of an increase in the amount of amniotic fluid.

Which of the following rashes is caused by the same infectious agent that accounts for the ultrasound findings in this patient?

    A. Grouped tender vesicles around the mouth and nose
    B. Numerous papules and vesicles on an erythematous base in addition to other lesions that have crusted
    C. A vesicular rash following a thoracic dermatome
    D. A diffuse macular rash with fine raised punctate lesions giving the skin a rough texture
    E. Bright red erythema of the cheeks that spares the perioral, nasal, and periorbital area, associated with a fine erythematous macular rash on the upper extremities

476.

A 4-month-old girl presents to the emergency room with a history of poor feeding, constipation, and decreased activity. Her mother reports that she "was fine" during a well-child examination 1 week earlier, at which time she received her scheduled immunizations. She normally takes 6 ounces of a commercial formula with each feeding in addition to rice cereal twice daily. On physical exam she is afebrile but appears lethargic. When examined her cry is weak. She is also noted to have bilateral ptosis and poor head control.

Which of the following is the most likely cause of the presenting signs and symptoms in this patient?

    A. Ingestion of *Clostridium botulinum* spores
    B. Adverse reaction to pertussis vaccine
    C. Non-accidental trauma—"shaken baby"
    D. Poliomyelitis
    E. Bacterial meningitis

477.

A 19-year-old college student who lives in the same suite with three other students presents to the emergency room with fever, malaise, and a rash. He is subsequently diagnosed with meningococcal meningitis.

Which of the following antimicrobial regimens is recommended for chemoprophylaxis of the index patient's roommates?

A. A single dose of rifampin 600 mg orally
B. A single dose of ciprofloxacin 500 mg orally
C. Azithromycin 500 mg orally on day 1 followed by 250 mg orally for 4 additional days
D. A single dose of amoxicillin 1 gram orally
E. Rifampin 600 mg orally once daily for 2 days

478.

An 8-year-old boy presents with a 2-day history of cough, nasal discharge, headache, and sore throat. Twice during the previous 6 weeks, following a positive throat culture for group A beta-hemolytic streptococci, he was treated with 250 mg of oral penicillin 2 times daily. His mother reports that her son completed a full 10 days of treatment on both occasions. On physical exam his temperature is 101.1° F. He has a prominent cough with clinical findings of bilateral conjunctival injection, clear nasal discharge, and erythematous enlarged tonsils. A throat culture is obtained, which is again positive for group A beta-hemolytic streptococci.

Which of the following is the most likely cause for the persistence of a positive throat culture in this patient despite the fact that he has recently completed two 10-day courses of antibiotic therapy?

A. Infection with penicillin-resistant group A beta-hemolytic streptococci
B. Inadequate length of antimicrobial therapy
C. Streptococcal carrier state
D. Inadequate dosage of antimicrobial therapy
E. Inappropriate choice of antimicrobial therapy

479.

The parents of a 7-year-old girl present with the concern that their daughter has had a rash for several days. By history the rash is non-pruritic. In addition they state that she has been "sleeping with her left eye partially opened." She had been well until 4–6 weeks ago, when she complained of fatigue, headache, and arthralgia. She was diagnosed with "a virus" and treated symptomatically at that time. On physical exam she has multiple annular erythematous lesions on the trunk and upper extremities. She is unable to close her left eye, and the left corner of her mouth droops.

Which of the following is the most likely cause of this patient's symptoms?

A. *Borrelia burgdorferi*
B. Herpes simplex virus
C. *Bartonella henselae*
D. *Rickettsia rickettsii*
E. *Ehrlichia chaffeensis*

480.

A 17-year-old male presents to the emergency room with complaints of abdominal pain associated with dizziness and shortness of breath, which began suddenly while he was lifting weights at a gym. The patient reports that during the preceding week he has felt fatigued and has had intermittent low-grade fever and myalgia. An emergent abdominal ultrasound shows evidence of splenic rupture.

Which of the following is most likely to be identified upon further evaluation of this patient?

A. Increased numbers of lymphocytes, including atypical lymphocytes, on peripheral smear
B. Thrombocytopenia
C. Elevated PT/PTT and bleeding time
D. Lymphoblasts with scant cytoplasm, condensed nuclear chromatin, and indistinct nucleoli on peripheral smear
E. Mature small lymphocytes associated with numerous "smudge" cells on peripheral smear

481.

A 4-year-old boy is admitted to the intensive care unit with altered mental status, fever, and rash. Cerebrospinal fluid cultures are positive for *Streptococcus pneumoniae*. Although initially very ill, he survives and is steadily improving. During a meeting to discuss discharge planning and follow-up, his parents inquire about potential long-term sequelae of his infection.

Which of the following represents the most common complication in children who survive an episode of bacterial meningitis?

A. Mental retardation
B. Seizures
C. Hearing loss
D. Spasticity and/or paresis
E. Panhypopituitarism

482.

A 3-year-old girl presents with a 24-hour history of an enlarging erythematous lesion on her left cheek. She is an active child, but her parents deny any known trauma to the involved area. On physical examination she appears uncomfortable and is irritable. Her temperature is 102.3° F. An intensely erythematous, indurated, tense, 3 x 6 cm tender plaque with sharply demarcated borders is present on her left cheek. In addition, there is associated enlargement of both the submandibular and anterior cervical lymph nodes on the left.

Which of the following is the most likely cause of this lesion?

A. Group A beta-hemolytic streptococci
B. *Bartonella henselae*
C. Atypical *Mycobacterium* species
D. *Streptococcus pneumoniae*
E. Herpes simplex virus

483.

A 4-year-old girl, recently adopted from an orphanage in the Dominican Republic, is diagnosed with varicella. Her adoptive parents have healthy 14-month-old twins who have not yet received varicella vaccine.

Which of the following choices describes the most appropriate intervention to prevent varicella infection in the twins?

A. Immediately begin oral acyclovir for a total of 10 days.
B. Administer varicella zoster immune globulin within 3–5 days following exposure.
C. Administer varicella vaccine within 24 hours following exposure in addition to oral acyclovir for a total of 14 days.
D. Administer varicella vaccine within 3–5 days following exposure.
E. Begin oral acyclovir if and when varicella lesions develop in one or both twins.

484.

An 18-year-old male presents complaining that he has noticed a tender "lump in his groin" that has progressively become larger and more tender over the last week. He reports generalized malaise, lethargy, and subjective fever but denies associated dysuria, frequency, urethral discharge, or recent trauma. He does report that, soon after returning from a cruise to the Caribbean, he noticed "five or six" small non-tender "pimples" on his penis, which he blamed on "getting sand in his bathing suit." Upon further questioning, he does share that he had sexual intercourse with several different women who "lived on the islands." On physical exam a very tender 2.5 x 3.5 cm inguinal lymph node is present in the right inguinal area.

Which of the following is the most appropriate treatment for this patient?

A. Ciprofloxacin 500 mg PO twice a day for 10 days
B. Trimethoprim-Sulfamethoxazole 160mg/800 mg PO twice a day for 10 days
C. Valacyclovir 1,000 mg PO twice a day for 2 weeks
D. Penicillin 500 mg PO twice a day for 2 weeks
E. Doxycycline 100 mg PO twice a day for 3 weeks

485.

A term female infant weighing 7 pounds, 6 ounces is transported to the normal newborn nursery following an uneventful delivery. During review of maternal prenatal records, it is noted that the infant's mother is hepatitis B surface antigen (HBsAg) positive.

Which of the following outlines the most appropriate intervention to lessen the risk that this infant will become infected by the hepatitis B virus?

A. Administer hepatitis B vaccine (HBV) as soon as possible followed by an additional vaccine dose at 1, 2, and 6 months of age.
B. Administer HBV and hepatitis B immune globulin (HBIG) as soon as possible followed by additional doses of both products at 2 and at 6 months of age.
C. Administer HBV and HBIG as soon as possible followed by additional doses of HBV at 2 and at 6 months of age.
D. Administer HBIG as soon as possible and at both 2 and 6 months of age.
E. Administer HBIG monthly until the infant becomes seronegative for HBsAg.

486.

A 14-year-old female presents with a 3-day history of fever and chills associated with bilateral wrist pain, right hand pain, and pain in the third, fourth, and fifth fingers of the left hand. Her temperature is 102° F. She has slight swelling and pain on movement of both wrists, her right hand, and all fingers of her left hand. She is also noted to have scattered 5–10 mm discrete, painful macules and maculopapular lesions over the upper extremities, including the palms. Several of the skin lesions are also petechial in nature. Laboratory results following initial evaluation of this patient include a positive blood culture.

Which of the following is the most likely organism associated with the positive blood culture?

A. *Staphylococcus aureus*
B. *Shigella sonnei*
C. *Borrelia burgdorferi*
D. *Neisseria gonorrhoeae*
E. *Salmonella typhi*

487.

A 2-year-old girl presents with a history of "hoarseness." Her mother goes on to state that her daughter's symptoms have continued to worsen over the last several months. She was evaluated 1 week ago in an emergency room and discharged home with the diagnosis of "croup." She has also been hospitalized twice for reactive airway disease. On physical examination she is afebrile with normal vital signs. A lateral x-ray of the airway shows a 1.8 x 2.7 cm localized, lobulated soft tissue mass on the posterior wall of the hypopharynx.

Which of the following is the most likely cause of this patient's radiological findings?

A. *Haemophilus influenzae* type b
B. Human papillomavirus Type 6
C. *Streptococcus pyogenes*
D. Viridans streptococci
E. Parainfluenza Type 1

488.

A mother who is hepatitis B surface antigen (HBsAg) positive wishes to breastfeed her newborn son. He was born at term via spontaneous vaginal delivery without complications.

Which of the following represents the most appropriate recommendation for infant feeding when the mother is HBsAg positive?

A. Breastfeeding is contraindicated when the mother is HBsAg positive.
B. Breastfeeding must be delayed for 7 days following administration of HBIG and HBV in the newborn nursery.
C. Breastfeeding must be delayed until the infant has received HBIG and HBV in the newborn nursery and a second HBV at one month of age.
D. Breastfeeding must be delayed for 24 hours following administration of two times the usual recommended dose for HBIG.
E. There is no need to delay initiation of breastfeeding.

489.

Identify the following organism:

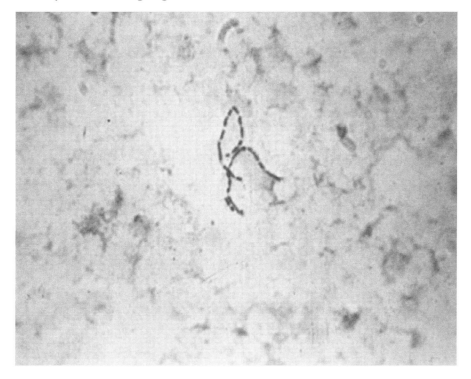

A. *Treponema pallidum*
B. *Chlamydia trachomatis*
C. *Chlamydophila pneumoniae*
D. *Haemophilus ducreyi*
E. *Klebsiella granulomatis* (formerly *Calymmatobacterium granulomatosis*)

490.

You receive a phone call from a mother of a 7-year-old African-American male whom you saw earlier in the week. By reviewing his chart, you note that you saw him 4 days ago and diagnosed him with chicken pox. At that time, when you examined him, he had had the lesions for 2 days. He was febrile with multiple varicella lesions, had slight congestion, but otherwise the exam was OK. He has been very healthy, and immunizations were up-to-date with the exception of varicella vaccine.

The reason the mother is calling today is her son is still running a 103° F fever and just doesn't seem to be getting better.

Which of the following is the best thing to tell her?

    A. Bring him in right away for evaluation and lab tests.
    B. You will call in famciclovir right away.
    C. Give him acetaminophen.
    D. This is a normal progression of the disease.
    E. He needs the varicella vaccine immediately.

491.

A 2-year-old from a daycare program in your area presents for evaluation. Yesterday her mother received word that 2 children in the daycare have been diagnosed with invasive *Haemophilus influenzae* type b; one of the cases was meningitis and the other was a buccal cellulitis. Your patient is up-to-date on all of her immunizations.

Based on this history, which of the following do you recommend?

    A. Only children in the daycare not up-to-date with their *H. influenzae* vaccines should receive prophylaxis.
    B. All children in the daycare should receive rifampin prophylaxis.
    C. Your patient, all other attendees, and all adults working in the daycare should receive rifampin prophylaxis.
    D. Only adults in the daycare should receive rifampin prophylaxis.
    E. Only non-up-to-date children and all adults should receive rifampin prophylaxis.

492.

A 2-year-old in daycare presents for evaluation. Today her mother learned that a case of meningococcal meningitis has occurred in one of the adults working at the center. None of the children are ill, and none of the other adults working at the center are ill.

Which of the following do you recommend?

    A. Observe the children and adults closely; if a 2nd case occurs then prophylax.
    B. Only the children need to be prophylaxed currently.
    C. Only the adults need to be prophylaxed currently.
    D. Counsel the parents of the children that if they are concerned, you can prophylax now—otherwise, it is safe to wait.
    E. Your patient and all children, as well as adult workers, who have had close contact with the infected index case should be prophylaxed with appropriate antibiotics.

493.

An 8-year-old boy presents with the following rash on his face:

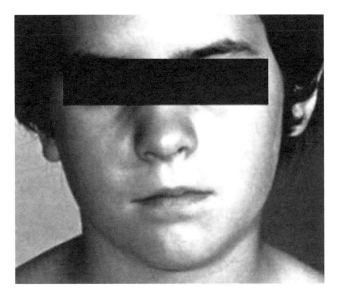

His teacher at school is pregnant.

Which of the following do you recommend as far as his returning to school?

    A. Wait until the rash is crusted over and then he may safely return to school.
    B. Wait 7 days after rash has appeared before he may return to school.
    C. Wait 5 days after rash has appeared before he may return to school.
    D. He may return to school now.
    E. He may return to school in 2 days.

494.

A 3-year-old in a daycare setting broke out with chickenpox this morning. He is doing clinically well and has few lesions.

Which of the following accurately states when he can return to daycare?

    A. The 4th day after onset of the rash, regardless of the stage of lesions
    B. The 6th day after onset only if no new lesions exist
    C. When all lesions are dried and crusted
    D. 10 days after onset
    E. 3 days after onset of the rash

495.

A 30-year-old nurse working in your immunization clinic develops herpes zoster in an 8th thoracic dermatome. Her only complaint is itching. Her Med/Peds physician places her on valacyclovir, and she asks about returning to work.

Which of the following is correct with regard to when she may return to work?

A. She must wait until 6 days after the appearance of the rash or until all of the lesions are crusted over.
B. She must wait until all of the lesions are crusted over.
C. As long as the lesions are kept covered by her clothes, she may return to work now.
D. She can return to work after she has been on the medication for 48 hours.
E. She can return to work in 10 days.

496.

Which of the following are routes for spread of infection in daycare settings or schools?

A. Fecal-oral
B. Respiratory
C. Contact with infected skin
D. Contact with blood, urine, or body secretions
E. All of the choices are possible routes

497.

A 9-year-old is diagnosed with measles infection. She is dehydrated and requires hospitalization for intravenous fluid therapy.

Which of the following is the appropriate isolation for her?

A. Private room, positive air-pressure ventilation, masks at all times, standard precautions
B. Private room, negative air-pressure ventilation, masks only if entrant into room is measles-antibody negative, standard precautions
C. Private room, negative air-pressure ventilation, masks at all times, standard precautions
D. Private room, standard precautions adequate
E. Private room, positive air-pressure ventilation, masks only if entrant into room is measles-antibody negative, standard precautions

498.

A 15-year-old male is bitten by his brother. The wound is to the hand and occurred 3 hours ago. This patient had his last tetanus immunization at age 11. His brother does not appear to have rabies. The patient is allergic to clindamycin.

Which of the following do you recommend?

A. Start amoxicillin-clavulanate.
B. Start trimethoprim-sulfamethoxazole.
C. Start trimethoprim-sulfamethoxazole and ciprofloxacin (since clindamycin allergic).
D. Start ciprofloxacin (since clindamycin allergic).
E. No antibiotics are necessary.

499.

A 13-year-old boy found a tick on his leg after hiking in the Colorado Rocky Mountains. His father calls and is concerned. You explain to him that he should remove the tick and that if the tick has been on less than 24 hours, there is little risk of transmission of disease.

Which of the following is the best method to remove a tick?

A. Use a lighted match to cause the tick to move and then remove the tick.
B. Squeeze the body of the tick tightly and pull it out.
C. Squeeze the head of the tick tightly and pull it out.
D. Grasp with a fine tweezer close to the skin and remove by gently pulling the tick straight out without twisting motions.
E. Grasp with a fine tweezer close to the skin and remove by gently pulling the tick with a twisting motion.

500.

A 17-year-old male presents after visiting his dentist earlier today. He was noted to have a dental abscess and required a tooth extraction. His dentist noted that he has a draining sinus tract.

PAST MEDICAL HISTORY: Significant only for dental caries for 3 years
SOCIAL HISTORY: Senior at local high school; B student
Smokes 1 pack/day of cigarettes
Reports no alcohol use
FAMILY HISTORY: Non-contributory
REVIEW OF SYSTEMS: Fever for 2 days
Cough present for a few days

PHYSICAL EXAMINATION:
BP 110/70, P 100, RR 20, Temp 102° F

HEENT: PERRLA, COMI
TM's Clear
Throat: Draining lesion noted from right molar with tract extending near buccal area
Heart: RRR without murmurs, rubs, or gallops
Lungs: Clear
Abdomen: Benign

LABORATORY: Gram stain shows beaded, branched, Gram-positive bacilli in the pus. Pathology notes "sulfur" granules.

Which of the following is the most likely organism?

A. *Actinomyces israelii*
B. *Streptococcus pneumoniae*
C. *Neisseria gonorrhea*
D. *Bacillus anthracis*
E. *Corynebacterium diphtheriae*

501.

A 12-year-old boy presents with a red-eye (see below). He had been swimming at the local pool 3 days ago. Initially his mother thought it was just the chlorine, but he woke up with "crust" in his eyes. She has called around, and 4 other children from that day at the pool now have the same red eye symptoms.

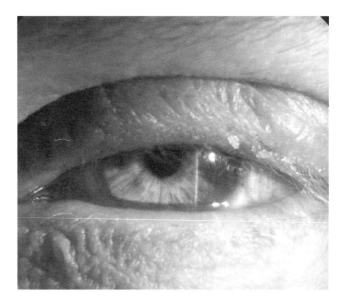

What is the most likely etiology?

A. *Streptococcus pneumoniae*
B. *Haemophilus influenzae*
C. Herpes simplex virus
D. Adenovirus
E. *Neisseria species*

502.

A 15-year old female living in Louisiana presents for evaluation. It is summer and she has frequent mosquito bites. She presents today with a complaint of headache and mild low-grade fever. She has vomited once today. She denies photophobia or other symptoms. Other kids in her neighborhood have had similar symptoms for several days. She has mild nuchal rigidity. You decide to perform a lumbar puncture.

Lumbar puncture results:
    WBC CSF 110 cells with 100% lymphocytes
    CSF protein 80 mg/dL
    CSF glucose 90 mg/dL

She recovers without incident.

Which of the following was the most likely etiology of her infection?

A. Herpes simplex virus
B. A bacteria
C. A fungus
D. An arbovirus
E. *Mycoplasma*

503.

A 30-year-old woman with negative past medical history presents to your Med/Peds colleague with a 1-week history of pain in her knees, wrists, and hands. She has been afebrile and has not had a rash. She lives in New Lyme, Connecticut. You had just recently seen her 8-year-old son with an erythematous rash that was on his face and arms. His rash got worse if he took a warm bath or was out in the sun. He also was afebrile.

Physical examination: Essentially normal except for her wrists and hands, which are moderately tender. No effusions of the joints are noted. She has no conjunctivitis or scleral changes on examination.

Which of the following is the likely etiology for both of their aliments?

A. Human herpesvirus 6
B. Parvovirus B19
C. Measles
D. *Borrelia burgdorferi*
E. *Neisseria gonorrhoeae*

504.

A 14-year-old is in her 32nd week of pregnancy. She presents to her obstetrician with fever and myalgias without any localizing symptoms. She denies any other problems. Her OB sends her to you for evaluation.

PAST MEDICAL HISTORY: 1st pregnancy; no problems until now
SOCIAL HISTORY: Doesn't smoke or drink
                         Attends 9th grade
FAMILY HISTORY: Non-contributory

PHYSICAL EXAMINATION: Normal (well, except for the large uterus at age 14!) except for a temperature of 102.5° F

LABORATORY:
   WBC: 12,000/mm^3; 70% neutrophils, 10% bands
   Urinalysis is normal
   Blood cultures are growing a Gram-positive diphtheroid-like organism

Which of the following is the most appropriate antibiotic for this organism?

A. Intravenous ceftriaxone
B. Intravenous clindamycin
C. Intravenous gentamicin
D. Intravenous penicillin G or ampicillin
E. Oral penicillin or amoxicillin

505.

An 8-year-old girl with otitis media is treated with an oral antibiotic and develops diarrhea. It is persistent and cultures are negative. A *C. difficile* toxin assay is sent on her stool and is positive. You treat the patient with metronidazole. She returns 2 weeks later with diarrhea again due to *C. difficile*.

Which of the following do you do now?

A. Treat with oral vancomycin.
B. Treat again with metronidazole.
C. Treat with oral vancomycin and clindamycin.
D. Treat with clindamycin.
E. Do not treat with antibiotics.

506.

Which of the following is the most common bacterium recovered from breast abscesses in newborns?

A. *Staphylococcus aureus*
B. *E. coli*
C. *Streptococcus pyogenes*
D. *Listeria monocytogenes*
E. *Streptococcus agalactiae*

507.

How does late-onset neonatal infection with *Listeria monocytogenes* present?

A. Meningitis
B. Pneumonia
C. Sepsis
D. UTI
E. Skin abscess

508.

Which of the following is true about pertussis in the newborn?

A. Because of maternal antibody, most newborn infants are immune to pertussis.
B. Most newborn infants are susceptible to pertussis.
C. Infants are immune if their mothers are up-to-date on their immunizations.
D. Infants are immune if their mothers had pertussis as a child.
E. Infants are immune if their mothers are up-to-date on their immunization or their mothers had pertussis as a child.

509.

Which of the following is true regarding neonatal tetanus?

A. Maternal antibodies are protective.
B. It occurs commonly in the United States in infants born to unimmunized mothers.
C. It occurs commonly in the United States in infants born to intravenous drug abusing mothers.
D. It occurs commonly in hypocalcemic babies.
E. It occurs commonly in babies who are immunocompromised.

510.

A 16-year-old girl with a negative past medical history presents to you with a 1-week history of pain in her left knee. She has had a low-grade fever and notes that she had a round "ring-like" rash 5 months ago. She lives in Massachusetts and regularly hikes in the woods.

PHYSICAL EXAMINATION: Essentially normal except for her left knee, which is moderately tender with an effusion. No effusions of other joints are noted. She has no conjunctivitis or scleral changes on examination. No rash is noted.

You send laboratory studies that are pending.

Which of the following is the best treatment?

A. Doxycycline 100 mg bid x 21 days
B. Ceftriaxone 2 grams IV x 21 days
C. Cefixime 400 mg x 1 dose
D. Erythromycin 500 mg qid x 21 days
E. Ciprofloxacin 500 mg bid x 7–10 days until afebrile

511.

A 16-year-old who lives on a farm comes to your office with a 2-week history of non-productive cough with fever. Additionally he has had sore throat and hoarseness associated with these symptoms. He has not had diarrhea or chills. He owns a pet cockatoo and several parakeets. He "chews" but doesn't smoke.

PAST MEDICAL HISTORY: Negative
SOCIAL HISTORY: Lives with his parents on their farm

PHYSICAL EXAMINATION: Vitals are normal except for a temperature of 100.8° F

HEENT:	PERRLA, EOMI
	Sclera anicteric
	Throat: red and inflamed; no exudates
Neck:	Supple
Heart:	RRR without murmurs, rubs, or gallops
Lungs:	Fine crackles heard at the right lung base; scattered wheezing
Abdomen:	Bowel sounds present
	No hepatosplenomegaly
Extremities:	No cyanosis, clubbing, or edema
Skin:	No rash

LABORATORY:

Leukocyte count:	12,000/mm^3; 60% neutrophils, 25% lymphocytes, 8% monocytes, 2% eosinophils
ESR:	57 mm/hr
TB Skin test:	0 mm
CXR:	Patchy infiltrate in the right lower lobe

Based on his age and physical findings, which of the following organisms is most likely to be causing his illness?

A. *Chlamydophila pneumoniae*
B. *Chlamydophila psittaci*
C. *Legionella pneumoniae*
D. *Coxiella burnetii*

512.

You diagnose diarrhea in a 10-year-old patient. The diarrhea is bloody in character.

For which of the following organisms would you <u>not</u> treat with antibiotics?

A. *Salmonella*
B. *Shigella*
C. *Campylobacter*
D. *C. difficile*
E. Ameba

513.

A 4-year-old with a recent history of otitis media treated with amoxicillin presents with a 4-hour history of severe headache, nausea, and vomiting and is now lethargic.

PAST MEDICAL HISTORY: Negative except for recent otitis 2 weeks ago; did not take all of her amoxicillin; stopped after 4 days

FAMILY HISTORY: Non-contributory

PHYSICAL EXAMINATION: T 102.6° F, P 110

HEENT:	PERRLA, EOMI
	Disc sharp
	TM's Clear
	Throat Clear
Neck:	Mild nuchal rigidity
Heart:	RRR without murmurs
Lungs:	Scattered crackles throughout; greatest in left lower lobe
Abdomen:	Benign
Extremities:	Normal
Neuro:	Lethargic
	No papilledema
	Cranial nerves tested intact
	No focal deficits

LABORATORY:

WBC:	20,000/mm^3; 76% segs, 10% bands
Electrolytes:	Normal
CSF WBC:	3,000/mm^3; 95% neutrophils
CSF glucose:	20 mg/dL (serum glucose 100 mg/dL)
CSF Protein:	176 mg/dL
CSF gram stain:	Loaded with neutrophils and a few gram-positive lancet shaped diplococci

Which of the following is the best antibiotic choice for her?

A. Ceftazidime alone
B. Vancomycin alone
C. Ampicillin and ceftazidime
D. Ceftriaxone and vancomycin
E. Penicillin

514.

A 14-year-old male with non-insulin dependent diabetes mellitus is seen in your office because of severe pain and tenderness of his right ear. He has been doing well before this.

SOCIAL HISTORY: Lives with his parents
                    Doesn't smoke or drink

PHYSICAL EXAMINATION:
BP 130/70, P 100, RR 20, Temp 103° F

HEENT:	PERRLA, EOMI
	TM's: Examination extremely painful and shows marked edema, erythema, and purulent material in the external auditory canal
	External ear is markedly swollen
	Throat: Clear
Neck:	Supple; no meningismus
Heart:	RRR without murmurs, rubs, or gallops
Lungs:	CTA
Abdomen:	Benign
Extremities:	No cyanosis, clubbing, or edema

Which of the following is the most likely etiology of his draining ear?

    A. *Staphylococcus aureus*
    B. *Streptococcus pneumoniae*
    C. *Pseudomonas aeruginosa*
    D. *Candida albicans*
    E. *Streptococcus diabeticus*

515.

Ted Nougat is an 8-year-old boy who comes to you with a 1-week history of fever, chills, and left eye conjunctivitis with an associated pre-auricular lymph node. He reports that he was well until this episode. He lives at home with a dog and 3 kittens. None of the pets have been ill.

PAST MEDICAL HISTORY: Negative
SOCIAL HISTORY: Dad is a veterinarian. The son spends time at dad's office and was recently bitten by a turtle and a rabbit.

PHYSICAL EXAMINATION: Besides the lymph node and the non-purulent conjunctivitis, everything else is normal.

He is started on oral cephalexin (Keflex®). He returns 3 days later with no improvement. A surgery colleague sees him and performs a biopsy, which shows necrotizing granuloma without organism. Acid-fast stains are negative.

Which of the following is the most likely organism responsible?

    A. *Borrelia burgdorferi*
    B. *Bartonella henselae*
    C. Herpes simplex I virus
    D. *Staphylococcus aureus*, methicillin resistant
    E. *Aeromonas hydrophilia*

516.

A 12-year-old male presents with a 3-day history of fever, malaise, and myalgias. He recently returned from a trip to Missouri, where he reports being bitten by a tick approximately 10 days ago. He was there on a fishing trip (he did quite well—20 lbs of fresh trout of which he brings you 2 of his best filets). He is healthy otherwise and reports that he was doing well.

PAST MEDICAL HISTORY:	Negative
SOCIAL HISTORY:	Lives with his mom and dad who are medical publishers
FAMILY HISTORY:	Negative

REVIEW OF SYSTEMS: No rash
No joint manifestations
No conjunctivitis
No lymphadenopathy

PHYSICAL EXAMINATION:
BP 120/70, P 100, RR 18, Temp 103° F

HEENT:	PERRLA, EOMI
	TM's clear
	Throat: clear
Neck:	Supple
Heart:	RRR without murmurs, rubs, or gallops
Lungs:	CTA
Abdomen:	Bowel sounds present; no hepatomegaly; spleen tip 2 cm below left costal margin
Extremities:	No cyanosis, clubbing, or edema

LABORATORY:
WBC:	2,200/mm^3; 60% polys, 20% bands
Hemoglobin:	12.5 mg/dL
Platelets:	140,000/mm^3
AST:	150 IU/L
ALT:	140 IU/L

Based on your history, physical, and laboratory values, which of the following is the most likely etiology?

A. Tularemia
B. Ehrlichiosis
C. Histoplasmosis
D. Blastomycosis
E. Lyme Disease

NEPHROLOGY

517.

A 7-year-old male with known minimal change disease nephropathy associated with 8.5 grams of proteinuria per day presents with increasing cough, shortness of breath, fever, and malaise of 6-hours duration. He has a BP of 106/78, pulse 96, temp of 39° C (102.2° F) and O_2 saturation of 91% on room air. His physical exam is notable for a normal cardiac exam, except for a 1/6 systolic ejection murmur, wheezes, and crackles at the bases of both lungs; a soft abdomen; and severe lower extremity edema—but with no leg pain or tenderness. Initial labs are essentially normal except for an albumin of 1.5 mg/dL and an elevated WBC of 17,000. A standard ECG is normal.

Which study is most appropriate to perform next and likely to confirm the diagnosis of the cause of his shortness of breath?

A. Duplex sonography of both lower extremities
B. Serial CK-MBs and troponin
C. Chest x-ray and sputum culture
D. CT angiography of the chest
E. Right-sided ECG

518.

Which of the following factors is <u>least</u> likely to contribute to the development of acute renal failure in a patient chronically treated with an angiotensin converting enzyme inhibitor (ACEI)?

A. Bilateral renal artery stenosis
B. Congestive heart failure with a known left ventricular ejection fraction of about 15%
C. Concomitant use of vancomycin intravenously
D. Severe gastroenteritis
E. Daily use of ibuprofen for juvenile inflammatory arthritis

519.

A 6-year-old boy with Fanconi syndrome from oculocerebrorenal syndrome (Lowe syndrome) is admitted with severe lower abdominal pain and hematuria. His exam is remarkable for a BP of 135/86, pulse 116, temperature of 38° C (100.0° F), and a respiratory rate of 28. His abdominal exam reveals no masses or point tenderness, and his rectal evaluation is also unremarkable. He does writhe intermittently throughout your history and physical.

Which of the following diagnostic tests would most likely lead to an accurate diagnosis?

A. A helical CT scan of the abdomen and pelvis
B. An exploratory laparotomy
C. A diagnostic abdominal tap
D. A liver function panel
E. Hepatic viral serologies

520.

A 14-year-old patient presents with a rapidly rising creatinine 2 years after an uncomplicated living-related kidney transplant. She has been eating and drinking well. She has a known history of mild chronic allograft nephropathy and a baseline creatinine of 1.7. Over the last six months, this level has risen to 2.6 and her blood pressure control has also worsened, now with a value of 190/110 mmHg. Her physical exam is otherwise unremarkable. She appears euvolemic, her urine output has been good, and the urinalysis is completely normal. She has a normal transplant ultrasound and CBC.

Which of the following diagnoses is most likely with this presentation?

    A. Acute cellular rejection
    B. Transplant renal artery stenosis
    C. Obstruction
    D. Hemolytic uremic syndrome
    E. Intravascular volume depletion

521.

A 17-year-old boy with known autosomal dominant polycystic kidney disease (PKD) has had a first episode of bleeding and painful cyst. You have treated him as an inpatient with IV hydration and pain medications. Since he is a new transfer to your care, you counsel him that he may suffer a number of non-renal complications from his PKD.

Which of the following complications should you inform him of with regard to his PKD?

    A. Diverticulosis
    B. Mitral valve prolapse
    C. Intracranial aneurysms
    D. Recurrent flank pain
    E. All of the answers are non-renal complications of PKD

522.

A 17-year-old boy with known autosomal dominant polycystic kidney disease (PKD) presents to the emergency room with symptoms suggestive of a urinary tract infection.

While awaiting results of the urine culture, which of the following antibiotics is the best initial empiric treatment?

    A. Ampicillin IV
    B. Trimethoprim/sulfamethoxazole
    C. Gentamicin
    D. Penicillin G IM

523.

Which of the following is <u>least</u> likely with the following ingestions?

A. Aspirin overdose and metabolic alkalosis
B. Methanol and visual changes
C. Aspirin overdose and tinnitus
D. Lithium and polyuria
E. Ethylene glycol and calcium oxalate crystals in the urine

524.

Which of the following is most likely to cause <u>spurious</u> hyperkalemia (pseudohyperkalemia)?

A. Thrombocytosis
B. Leucopenia
C. Metabolic acidosis
D. Rhabdomyolysis
E. Hyperlipidemia

525.

Which of the following is (are) <u>not</u> a feature(s) distinctive of Type 1 (distal) renal tubular acidosis compared to other RTAs?

A. Kidney stones
B. Hypokalemia
C. Nephrocalcinosis
D. Fanconi syndrome and hyperkalemia

526.

A 5-year-old girl with spina bifida is being evaluated for hematuria. She has a history of urinary tract infections, but she has been healthy for the past 6 months and is not on any new medications. She has no family history of kidney disease. On physical exam, her blood pressure is 92/60, and the rest of her exam is consistent with spina bifida but otherwise unremarkable. On further evaluation, you note 10–15 RBCs/HPF but no casts or crystals. She has no proteinuria; the serologic evaluation, including complements, ANCA, and ANA, are all within normal limits. A urine calcium-to-creatinine ratio is 0.9. The ultrasound shows only one apparently normal-appearing kidney without evidence of obstruction. A urine culture returns with no growth.

Which of the following is the best management strategy at this time?

A. Start oxybutynin to prevent bladder spasms.
B. Push fluids, limit sodium intake, and maintain regular follow-up and vigilance for kidney stones.
C. Hospitalize and biopsy.
D. Empirically treat with antibiotics.
E. Perform an IVP or helical CT scan.

527.

An 8-year-old girl has advanced chronic kidney disease due to grade 5 vesicoureteral reflux. She continues to have recurrent infections and was hospitalized last month with an *E. coli* pyelonephritis. Her parents have refused corrective surgery. She takes a daily dose of trimethoprim-sulfamethoxazole as UTI prophylaxis. Her family history is notable for several paternal relatives with colon cancer, and her mother has diabetes mellitus Type 2. On physical exam, you note mild hypertension for age, and height and weight at approximately the 5th percentile for age. Her nephrologist, who saw her last week, has not referred her for transplantation but feels she will need dialysis in less than 6 months.

Which of the following would explain a delay in transplantation in this child?

A. She must grow a bit larger before she can be technically transplanted.
B. She has recurrent infections.
C. She must not be on TMP-SMX within 12 months of a transplant.
D. Her family history must be corrected.
E. She must be on dialysis before getting a transplant.

528.

A 15-year-old girl begins to experience recurrent headaches at the start of the volleyball season. Her school performance has been excellent, her menses are regular and not associated with many of these headaches, and she takes no over-the-counter medications or prescription drugs. She does have a family history of hypertension and Type 2 diabetes mellitus. On physical, her BP is 188/110 (her records indicate she has had a normal BP on prior visits), she is 50th percentile for height and 25th percentile for weight, and she has symmetric and strong pulses. Her cardiovascular exam is otherwise normal, with the exception of a faint bruit to the right of her umbilicus. Her lungs are clear; she has an otherwise unremarkable exam.

Which of the following diagnoses is most likely at this point?

A. Coarctation of the aorta
B. Essential hypertension
C. Cocaine use
D. Stress of academics and volleyball try-outs
E. Fibromuscular dysplasia

529.

Which of the following comorbidities is _not_ consistent with advanced chronic kidney disease?

A. Anemia
B. Psychosocial disruption
C. Volume-related hypertension
D. Hypokalemia
E. Growth delay

530.

A previously well 10-year-old boy is admitted with severe diarrhea. His physical exam is notable for very dry mucosa and a SBP in the low 80s. His abdomen is diffusely tender, but his physical exam is otherwise unremarkable. His labs are generally normal, with the exception of a creatinine of 1.8 mg/dL and a urine-specific gravity of 1.030 with an otherwise bland UA. In addition, you obtain urinary studies and estimate a fractional excretion of sodium (FENa) of less than 1%.

Which of the following diagnoses do these findings support?

A. HUS/TTP
B. Pre-renal azotemia
C. Acute tubular necrosis
D. Acute rejection
E. Minimal change disease

531.

Which of the following is true with regard to arterial blood gases?

A. There is no **full** compensation for primary acid-base disorders.
B. The generation of an anion gap is physiologically unlimited.
C. 1 mmol of generated acid may result in more than 1 mmol of bicarbonate.
D. All anions are accounted for in routine blood chemistries.
E. All of the answer options are false.

532.

A 4-year-old child is discovered to have microscopic hematuria on a dipstick during a well-child check when she complained of "stomach" pain. She is otherwise completely healthy, growing and developing normally, and has a normal physical. Several follow-up urinalyses continue to demonstrate microscopic hematuria without casts or crystals.

Which of the following would be the appropriate next step in evaluation?

A. Refer her for a diagnostic kidney biopsy.
B. Obtain a full set of serologies.
C. Check a random urine calcium-to-creatinine ratio.
D. Notify child protective services of your concern.
E. Check to see if her co-pay has gone up with the new contract.

533.

An obese, 17-year-old girl has been recently diagnosed with diabetes mellitus Type 2. You spend considerable time discussing weight loss, proper eating, and a healthy lifestyle.

In addition, to screen for microvascular disease and kidney disease in particular, which of the following is appropriate?

  A. You should screen for microalbuminuria now.
  B. You should wait 5 years before screening for microalbuminuria.
  C. The standard urine dip-stick is sufficient for screening for diabetic kidney disease.
  D. Focus on weight loss and deal with the kidneys later.
  E. An eye exam will suffice to check for all microvascular disease.

534.

Which of the following statements about aminoglycoside (AG)-associated nephrotoxicity is <u>not</u> true?

  A. There is typically a time lag of 7–10 days after the start of therapy before clinical evidence of ATN begins to occur.
  B. Nephrotoxicity is proportionate to the total dose of AG.
  C. Other nephrotoxic agents increase the risk of ATN.
  D. Coadministration of dopamine reduces the risk.
  E. Elevated trough levels increase risk of ATN.

535.

An 8-year-old girl presents to the emergency room with a 3-day history of an unrelenting headache. Associated symptoms include generalized malaise, lethargy, and decreased appetite. Her mother has also noted decreased urine output, which she attributes to her daughter's poor appetite. She has otherwise been well, except for the fact that she was recently treated for scabies. On physical examination, her blood pressure is 160/105. She appears lethargic and complains of abdominal pain. Although there are multiple papules and vesicular lesions that appear to be drying and fading, others are moist and crusted with an associated yellowish discharge. A urinalysis, obtained in part to assess the extent of dehydration, is positive for large numbers of red blood cells.

Which of the following laboratory findings is most likely to be identified upon further evaluation of this patient?

  A. Elevated levels of amylase and lipase
  B. Blood and urine cultures positive for *E. coli*
  C. Multiple calcium oxalate crystals in the urine
  D. Normal levels of C3 and CH50
  E. An elevated deoxyribonuclease (DNAse) B antibody level

536.

A 19-year-old male presents to his college infirmary because he noticed that his "urine was red." He smells strongly of alcohol and admits to "partying hard" during the previous two days while "rushing with his fraternity brothers." He also states that his "leg muscles have been sore" since he awakened after "passing out for the night." He denies any associated pain on urination or increased urinary frequency. His vital signs are stable. He is lethargic and belligerent on exam, but no specific abnormalities are evident. A urine sample is grossly red and heme-positive. Red blood cells are absent upon microscopic examination of the urine.

Which of the following laboratory findings is most likely to be identified upon further evaluation of this patient?

A. Elevated titers of Antistreptolysin O (ASO) antibodies
B. Uric acid crystals on microscopic examination of the urine
C. Increased urinary levels of delta-aminolevulinic acid and porphobilinogen
D. Hypercalcemia
E. Elevated levels of serum creatinine kinase

537.

The parents of a 6-year-old girl present with the concern that their daughter's hands and feet have become progressively "swollen" over the previous week. In addition, when she awoke on the day of presentation her "eyes were so swollen she could barely open them." She had previously been well and takes no daily medications. On physical examination, she has noticeable swelling of the hands and feet in addition to nontender bilateral periorbital edema. Her blood pressure is 84/52 and she is afebrile. She is irritable on exam with diffuse mild abdominal pain. Urinalysis is positive for 4+ protein and trace blood.

Which of the following laboratory findings is most likely to be present upon further evaluation of the patient?

A. A platelet count of 35,000
B. Creatinine of 4.2 mg/dL
C. Elevated urinary levels of homovanillic acid and vanillylmandelic acid (VMA)
D. Hemoglobin of 7.8 g/dL
E. Serum triglyceride of 310 mg/dL

538.

An 11-year-old girl presents with a 3-day history of dysuria. She reports no associated increase in urinary frequency, abdominal pain, or fever. The etiology of her symptoms is thought to be related to local irritation rather than a urinary tract infection, because the patient's mother reports that she will frequently take long bubble baths. However, urine is obtained as a precaution. The only abnormal finding on urine dipstick is 3+ (300–1000 mg/dL) protein.

Which of the following is the most appropriate next step in the evaluation of this patient?

A. Urine culture
B. Renal ultrasound
C. Timed 24-hour urine collection for protein
D. Urine calcium/creatinine ratio on the first morning void followed by a second urine calcium/creatinine ratio on an upright specimen
E. Urine protein/creatinine ratio on the first morning void followed by a second urine protein/creatinine ratio on an upright specimen

539.

A 3-year-old boy presents to the emergency room after his parents became concerned that he "looked pale and exhausted." He was evaluated about a week earlier for an episode of bloody diarrhea that followed 2 days of watery diarrhea, fever, vomiting, and abdominal pain. His parents were told that he "had a virus" and that the source of blood in his stool was from excessive skin irritation in the diaper area due to his frequent stools. Laboratory findings include a hemoglobin of 8.4 g/dL, leukocyte count of 31,000, platelet count of 35,000, and creatinine of 1.8 mg/dL.

Which of the following organisms is the most likely cause of this patient's illness?

A. *Escherichia coli*
B. *Salmonella typhi*
C. *Shigella flexneri*
D. *Clostridium difficile*
E. *Campylobacter jejuni*

540.

A 6-day-old male born by emergency cesarean section due to fetal distress after his mother was involved in an automobile accident is noted to have grossly bloody urine. His Apgar scores were 2/4/7. He currently requires mechanical ventilation and is also being treated for presumed sepsis. On physical examination, a mass in the right flank is noted.

Which of the following is the most likely etiology of this patient's clinical findings?

A. Hemolytic uremic syndrome
B. Hereditary nephritis (Alport syndrome)
C. Renal vein thrombosis
D. Autosomal recessive polycystic kidney disease
E. Ureteropelvic junction obstruction

541.

A 17-year-old male presents after discovering a "lump in his left testicle" while showering. He denies any associated trauma, pain, or dysuria. He has had several female sexual partners and uses a condom only sporadically. On physical exam, a painless cystic-like nodule located above the upper pole of the left testicle is identified on palpation. Additional evaluation indicates that the nodule transilluminates.

Which of the following is a likely component of this nodule?

A. Gram-negative intracellular diplococci
B. Sperm
C. Peritoneal fluid
D. Embryonic remnants of the müllerian ductal system
E. Neoplastic germ cells

542.

Which of the following is true regarding the use of a blood pressure cuff that covers 1/2 of the length of the upper arm?

A. This will likely give erroneously low readings.
B. This will likely give erroneously high readings.
C. This is an appropriate size for a child less than 25 kgs.
D. This is likely to cause constriction significant enough to cause pain and discomfort.
E. May show pulsus paradoxus.

543.

Which of the following is <u>not</u> true regarding angiotensin-converting enzyme (ACE) inhibitors?

A. Associated with angioedema
B. Likely to lower blood pressure in patients with renal artery stenosis
C. Able to prevent progressive renal dysfunction in patients with Type 1 diabetes mellitus
D. Responsible for increased renin in hypertensive subjects
E. Frequently stopped for hyperkalemia

544.

A 17-year-old female presents with altered mental status. No medical history is available. Other than being stuporous, her exam is unremarkable with normal vital signs, no orthostasis, no edema, and without focal findings. Her serum sodium is 104 mEq/L (very low!), creatinine 0.6 mg/dL (normal), U_{Na+} 8 mEq/L (**low**), and Uosm is 90 mOsm/kg H_2O (**low**).

Which of the following is true?

A. Treatment should start with hypertonic saline.
B. Her total body sodium is approximately normal.
C. She has an excess of antidiuretic hormone.
D. Diuretic abuse should be suspected.
E. Water intoxication has been ruled out.

545.

A 19-year-old presents for evaluation of renal insufficiency and proteinuria. He has a 10-year history of diabetes and the recent onset of hypertension. He has had treatment for diabetic polyneuropathy and retinopathy within the past year. Exam shows eye and nerve abnormalities, blood pressure of 160/102 mmHg, and mild edema—but is otherwise normal. Labs demonstrate a sodium of 138, potassium of 4.0, chloride of 108, bicarbonate 20, creatinine 1.3, and BUN of 28 mg/dL. The blood sugar is 186 mg/dL, albumin 3.4g/dL. Urine shows a creatinine clearance of 40 mL/min and 3.4 g/day of protein.

Which of the following is the most appropriate treatment of his renal condition?

    A. Blood pressure reduction with a dihydropyridine
    B. Weight loss, blood sugar control, and low-salt diet
    C. Renal biopsy
    D. Enalapril
    E. Magnetic renal angiography

546.

Which of the following lab values are consistent with a child drinking ethylene glycol?

    A. Na 143, K 4.8, Cl 100, HCO_3-10, Serum creatinine 3.5, arterial pH 7.25
    B. Na 135, K 4.5, Cl 106, HCO_3-22, Serum creatinine 3.5, arterial pH 7.37
    C. Na 140, K 2.6, Cl 115, HCO_3-13, Serum creatinine 3.5, arterial pH 7.31
    D. Na 140, K 5.2, Cl 102, HCO_3-20, Serum creatinine 3.5, arterial pH 7.36
    E. Na 140, K 6.2, Cl 109, HCO_3-20, Serum creatinine 3.5, arterial pH 7.36

547.

A 5-year-old girl with unexplained gross and microscopic hematuria has a normal intravenous pyelogram as well as a normal ultrasound. All of her renal function tests are normal. This phenomenon is fairly common in children.

With which of the following is this common condition associated?

    A. Hypercalcemia
    B. Hypercalciuria
    C. Hyperkaluria
    D. Hyperphosphatemia
    E. Severe urethritis

548.

Which of the following is true about acute glomerulonephritis in childhood?

A. It is most common between 12 and 17 years of age.
B. It usually follows the onset of a streptococcal infection by 1 to 2 days.
C. It is generally associated with high complement levels.
D. Prednisone is the usual treatment.
E. It can occur with a normal urinalysis.

549.

A 5-year-old boy is discovered on routine physical to have dipstick-positive proteinuria (1+ to 2+ on various occasions). His physical examination is entirely normal. All other laboratory is also normal.

Which of the following is the appropriate next step?

A. Reassure and see the patient in follow-up next year.
B. Perform quantitative supine and upright urine protein testing.
C. Send the patient to a nephrologist for a kidney biopsy.
D. Culture the throat and urine for possible silent streptococcal infection.
E. Continue to check urine dipsticks for spontaneous resolution.

550.

A 10-month-old boy is in for a well-child check. His mother is concerned, because she usually only palpates one testicle.

In discussing this issue with her, which of the following is true?

A. Testes usually descend by 6 months, and if not by then, should have surgery before one year.
B. Retractile testes are at risk for seminoma and need surgical correction.
C. There is an increased risk for seminoma in ectopic testicles.
D. Orchiopexy is best performed before 10 years of age.
E. Cryptorchidism is associated with a lower IQ.

NERVOUS SYSTEM / NEUROLOGY

551.

A neonate presents with the findings below.

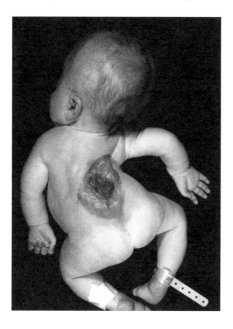

Which of the following abnormalities might you expect to see on an MRI of the brain?

A. Hydrocephalus
B. Chiari I malformation
C. Polymicrogyria
D. Porencephalic cyst

552.

A mother comes in with her child, who has been diagnosed with spina bifida.

Which of the following would be the risk of recurrence in the next sibling, should she decide to have another child?

A. Population risk
B. 4%
C. 10%
D. 25%

553.

A 13-year-old child comes in with a history of several weeks of increasing headaches and vomiting. He is afebrile and has no history of infection. His symptoms worsen with lying flat. He complains of double vision.

Which of the following cranial nerve abnormalities might you discover associated with this disease?

A. IV nerve palsy
B. VIII nerve palsy
C. VI nerve palsy
D. X nerve palsy

554.

Which of the following is the most common cause of cerebral palsy (CP)?

A. Perinatal asphyxia
B. Low birthweight/prematurity
C. Genetic abnormalities
D. Infection

555.

A 10-year-old child is brought in after being hit in the head with a hockey puck. He was not wearing a helmet. His mother reports that he had a period where he seemed fine but has since become lethargic and difficult to rouse. On examination you notice that he is difficult to rouse, has begun to posture, and one pupil is much larger than the other.

Which of the following might you find on CT?

A. Subdural hemorrhage
B. Intraparenchymal hemorrhage
C. Subgaleal hemorrhage
D. Epidural hemorrhage
E. Intraventricular hemorrhage

556.

A child comes in after having been sacked in a football game. He reports a brief period of amnesia around the event. His father reports that he may have lost consciousness. He currently has a headache and says that he is seeing double. His gait is ataxic. His CT scan of the head is normal.

Which of the following represents when he may return to sports?

A. One week after the injury
B. Two weeks after the injury
C. Two weeks after a normal neurological exam and no symptoms
D. One week after a normal neurological exam and no symptoms
E. Out for the season

557.

You are working in the newborn nursery and performing a well-baby check. On examination, you see this:

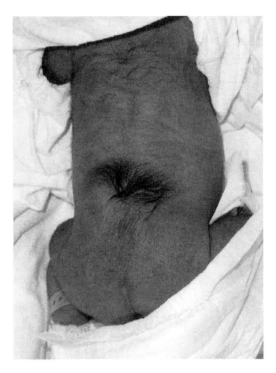

Which of the following abnormalities is <u>not</u> associated with this finding?

A. Syringomyelia
B. Diastematomyelia
C. Chiari I malformation
D. Tethered cord

558.

A child is reported to be having trouble paying attention at school. Her mother describes multiple brief periods of eyelid fluttering daily. An EEG shows 3 Hz spike-and-wave discharges.

Which of the following is the treatment of choice?

A. Carbamazepine
B. Phenytoin
C. Ethosuximide
D. Phenobarbital

559.

A child comes in with a large head and multiple café-au-lait spots. He has visual problems and is said to be doing poorly at school.

Which of the following is the mode of inheritance of his disease?

A. Autosomal dominant
B. Autosomal recessive
C. Trinucleotide repeat
D. Sporadic

560.

A 5-year-old child presents with nighttime episodes of facial twitching and difficulty talking. The episodes evolve into generalized shaking at times. He is developmentally normal.

Which of the following is the pattern you would expect to see on EEG?

A. 3 Hz spike and wave
B. 4–6 Hz polyspike and wave
C. Centrotemporal sharp waves
D. Occipital sharp waves

561.

A 17-year-old female presents to the emergency room after her mother found her on the bathroom floor "stiff, drooling, and uncontrollably shaking her arms and legs." Her mother denies any previous history of similar episodes or known seizures. She is otherwise well with the exception of "morning jerks," which have been diagnosed as "tics" related to her use of methylphenidate for attention deficit disorder (ADD). On further history, the patient's mother does express concern that her daughter's "tics are sometimes so severe that she has trouble getting ready for school in the morning." The "tics" are reported to be infrequent after the morning hours. An EEG, especially upon photic stimulation, is abnormal.

Which of the following describes the typical clinical course in such patients?

A. Continued progression of symptoms despite discontinuation of all stimulant medications for ADD
B. Periventricular calcifications on MRI of the brain
C. Effective control of subsequent seizures upon treatment with valproate
D. Onset of frequent and difficult-to-control seizures despite aggressive therapy with multiple anticonvulsants
E. Progressive symptoms of muscle wasting oftentimes associated with cardiomyopathy and early cardiac death

562.

A 12-year-old female with a history of a seizure disorder presents to the emergency room following a generalized tonic-clonic seizure estimated to have lasted for 20 minutes. The patient is lethargic but oriented to time, place, and person. She admits that she has not taken her anticonvulsant regularly, because she is "mad about having to take medicine every day." She also has a history of hypertension and scoliosis. Her blood pressure is 160/98. Physical examination is positive for axillary freckling and an abdominal bruit in the area of the left renal artery.

Which of the following physical findings is most likely to be identified upon additional examination of this patient?

A. A hypopigmented skin lesion on the anterior thigh
B. A congenital cataract
C. A "port wine" facial nevus in the ophthalmic distribution of the trigeminal nerve
D. Multiple hemangiomas
E. Numerous oval macular light brownish-tan lesions on the anterior and posterior trunk

563.

The parents of a 15-month-old girl present with concerns that their daughter's "seizures are not getting any better." She was placed on valproic acid following an emergency room visit about 6 weeks earlier. A head CT was reported as normal prior to discharge. Her parents confirm that they have been compliant with medication. Seizure activity is described as "repetitive head jerking while holding her head to one side." The patient initially appears well but, despite remaining alert, is noted to suddenly develop torticollis associated with head nodding and nystagmus. An emergent head MRI is normal.

Which of the following is the most appropriate next step in the treatment of this patient?

A. Discontinue valproic acid and begin phenytoin.
B. Continue valproic acid and add phenobarbital.
C. Continue valproic acid and add pyridoxine.
D. Discontinue valproic acid and begin carbamazepine.
E. Discontinue all anticonvulsant therapy.

564.

A 15-year-old female presents with her parents for a second opinion regarding "unrelenting foot and ankle pain" over a 4-week period, which seems to worsen with any attempt at exercise. During the last week she has been unable to tolerate sleeping with even a bed sheet touching her ankle. Several weeks prior to the onset of her pain, she sprained her ankle at soccer practice, but had to miss practice for only 2 days before returning. On exam her ankle is exquisitely tender and cool to touch. The ankle and foot are edematous, and appear bluish in color with decreased peripheral pulses and limited range of motion. A CBC, erythrocyte sedimentation rate (ESR), and complete metabolic panel are within normal limits. Plain radiographs of the foot and ankle show no evidence of fracture.

Which of the following is the most appropriate next step in the treatment of this patient?

 A. A nonsteroidal antiinflammatory agent (NSAID)
 B. A narcotic analgesic
 C. Immobilization
 D. Physical therapy
 E. Interarticular injection of corticosteroids

565.

During an evaluation for fever and fussiness, a 16-month-old girl is noted to have a generalized tonic-clonic seizure which lasts for 3–4 minutes. Immediately following the seizure, she is lethargic but appears to recognize her parents. She soon is "back to herself" according to her parents. Her temperature is 103.4° F. Other vital signs are normal. The right tympanic membrane is erythematous and bulging, but no other abnormalities are noted. Her father reports that he too had several "seizures" when he was a toddler.

In addition to treating her otitis media, which of the following is the most appropriate next step in the treatment of this patient?

 A. Obtain a CT scan of the head followed by, if the scan is normal, a lumbar puncture.
 B. Obtain an MRI of the head and, if normal, begin outpatient treatment with valproic acid.
 C. Administer a loading dose of phenobarbital, followed by admission to the hospital for observation and additional evaluation.
 D. Discharge the patient home, with outpatient follow-up in 24–48 hours.
 E. Begin treatment with ethosuximide.

566.

The parents of an 8-year-old girl express their frustration that their daughter's school performance has not improved since beginning methylphenidate for attention deficit disorder. Her grades continue to be poor, and her teacher is concerned that she often appears as if she is "staring into space with a blank look on her face." Compliance with medication has not been an issue, and side effects are denied. The patient herself is frustrated and appears to be motivated. As part of her exam she is asked to hyperventilate. Soon afterwards she is noted to have a brief episode of staring while rubbing her fingers together during which time she does not respond to questions. An EEG is ordered, and it is abnormal.

Which of the following medications is most effective in this type of seizure disorder?

 A. Ethosuximide
 B. Valproic acid
 C. Phenobarbital
 D. Carbamazepine
 E. Phenytoin

567.

An 11-year-old boy is transported to the emergency room after his mother found him to be unresponsive when she attempted to awaken him. He is febrile and difficult to arouse. Multiple petechial, purpuric, and ecchymotic lesions are noted on the trunk and extremities. Following stabilization, a lumbar puncture is performed. Gram stain of a CSF sample reveals numerous Gram-negative diplococci.

Which of the following is often identified in patients at increased risk for infection with the organism responsible for this meningitis?

- A. Terminal complement component deficiency
- B. Reducing substances in the urine
- C. Elevated serum ammonia levels
- D. Reed-Sternberg cells on bone marrow biopsy
- E. Glomerular hypercellularity with crescent formation on renal biopsy

568.

A 7-year-old boy is rushed to the emergency room after his parents found him "shaking all over" soon after he had gone to bed. He appeared well in the emergency room and complained only of being tired. Laboratory findings, including a urine drug screen and a head CT, were normal. He was discharged and told to follow up with a neurologist for a possible seizure disorder. Prior to the appointment he experienced 2 episodes of sudden difficulty swallowing, associated with facial numbness, drooling, and difficulty with speech. The patient has full recollection of both episodes and remembers "making grunting noises" and feeling like he "was choking."

Which of the following best describes the expected prognosis for this patient?

- A. He is likely to develop severe dementia by 40–50 years of age.
- B. Lifelong therapy with valproic acid will be required to adequately control seizure activity.
- C. He will experience more frequent and progressively worsening episodes of dysphagia and dysarthria and will likely require a gastronomy tube by his early 20s.
- D. He will develop difficult-to-treat motor and vocal tics within the next several years.
- E. Spontaneous regression of all symptoms will likely occur within the next several years.

569.

A 9-year-old girl presents with a 5-day history of lower back pain, which has recently become associated with complaints of "burning and stinging pain" shooting down her legs. In addition, she complains of significant pain when clothing comes in contact with her skin. Her parents have also noticed that she has been dragging her right leg when walking and has had several recent episodes of urinary incontinence. Three days prior to the onset of pain she was treated with azithromycin for presumed *Mycoplasma* pneumonia.

Which of the following findings will most likely be identified upon further evaluation of this patient?

A. Decreased levels of protein in cerebrospinal fluid
B. Positive blood culture for *Staphylococcus aureus*
C. Swelling of a segment of the spinal cord on MRI
D. Fracture of the pars interarticularis at L5 on bone scan
E. Anterior slippage of the L5 vertebral body on S1 on an oblique plain film

570.

A post-term 10-pound, 2-ounce male is born to an insulin-dependent diabetic mother following a difficult vaginal delivery. During initial evaluation in the newborn nursery, he is noted to have crepitance over the mid-portion of the right clavicle and isolated paralysis of the right hand. A brachial plexus injury is diagnosed.

Assuming that the injury does not improve over time, which of the following findings on physical examination is consistent with an injury that included damage to the T1 nerve root?

A. Anisocoria associated with heterochromia
B. Inability to contract the lower facial muscles on the right side, associated with the appearance of a "drooping" mouth
C. Loss of the nasolabial fold on the right
D. Inability of the right eye to move laterally beyond the midline
E. Corneal enlargement associated with excessive tearing and a corneal haze

571.

A 16-year-old female with a history of frequent migraine headaches and depression presents to the emergency room in an agitated and combative state. Just prior to presentation, her mother found her "vomiting and talking out of her head" in the bathroom. Her only chronic medications are zolmitriptan and fluoxetine. She appears confused and is obviously hallucinating, while both shivering and sweating profusely. Temperature is 103.4° F, heart rate is 130 beats/minute, and blood pressure is 155/105 mmHg. On neurological exam she is noted to have hyperreflexia and clonus and is incontinent of both stool and urine.

Which of the following is the most likely cause of this patient's symptoms?

A. Excess levels of serotonin
B. Hemorrhage due to an arteriovenous malformation
C. Heroin overdose
D. New onset diabetes mellitus presenting as diabetic ketoacidosis
E. Benzodiazepine overdose

572.

A 20-month-old girl presents for a health maintenance examination. Her parents report that she seems "clumsy" and is having greater difficulty feeding herself and grasping, transferring, and picking up toys than she did just a few months ago. They also express concern that she no longer puts 2 or more words together and has taken to pointing and grunting to express her needs and desires. Review of her previous records and growth charts shows no concerns about her growth and development, with the exception that her head circumference, including today's visit, has gradually decreased from the 55th to the 10th percentile. Throughout the encounter she is noted to frequently rub, tap, and/or squeeze her hands.

When compared to the general population, this patient is at increased risk of sudden death from which one of the following causes?

A. Cardiac arrhythmia
B. Intracerebral hemorrhage
C. Cerebral herniation
D. Thromboembolism
E. Aortic root dissection

573.

During a slit-lamp examination, a 7-year-old girl with a history of scoliosis and a seizure disorder is noted to have multiple oval yellowish-brown, dome-shaped papules that appear to project from the surface of the iris. Her father reports that he has been told by an ophthalmologist that he has similar appearing lesions.

Which of the following describes the associated chromosomal abnormality in patients with this disorder?

A. Trisomy 18
B. Monosomy X (45X)
C. A gene mutation on the long arm of chromosome 17
D. A gene deletion on the paternal copy of chromosome 15
E. A gene deletion on the maternally inherited chromosome 15

574.

A 15-year-old male presents to the ER complaining of weakness of both legs. He reports that he started to have a tingling sensation in his toes about a day ago. Next, he noticed a "foot drop" sensation developing. On awakening this morning, he had problems grasping objects and noted some weakness in his upper legs. He has had no fever, diplopia, dysphagia, or dyspnea. He had a "cold" 1 week prior to his current symptoms. He removed a tick from his waist about a week and a half ago. He eats home-grown vegetables and fruits that his grandmother cans for him back in West Virginia.

PAST MEDICAL HISTORY: Negative
IMMUNIZATIONS: Up-to-date

SOCIAL HISTORY: Attends 9th grade
                         Doesn't drink alcohol

FAMILY HISTORY: Negative

PHYSICAL EXAMINATION:
BP 120/76, RR 18, Temp 97.9° F, P 86

HEENT:	PERRLA, EOMI
	Discs sharp
	TMs clear
	Throat clear
Neck:	Supple
Heart:	RRR with I/VI systolic flow murmur
Lungs:	CTA
Abdomen:	Bowel sounds present; no hepatosplenomegaly
Extremities:	No cyanosis, clubbing, or edema
Neuro:	Symmetrical weakness of lower extremities—
	distal more affected than proximal muscles
	Bilateral foot drop
	Weakness of both hands noted
	Cranial Nerves II–XII are tested intact
	Sensory perception is normal
	Patellar and Achilles reflexes are absent bilaterally

Which of the following is the most likely diagnosis?

A. Botulism (food-borne)
B. Guillain-Barré syndrome
C. Poliomyelitis
D. Tick paralysis
E. Rabies

575.

A 16-year-old high school student is brought into the ER by his friends because they were unable to awaken him this morning. They are all staying at Mark's house, whose parents are out of town. They report that he has not had any alcohol and is a model student. During the past 2 to 3 days, however, they say that Mark has exhibited bizarre behavior and has been increasingly confused. He takes no medications, and his friends adamantly deny that he has ever used any type of illicit drug.

PAST MEDICAL HISTORY: Treated for gonorrhea 1 year ago
FAMILY HISTORY: Negative

PHYSICAL EXAMINATION:
T 102° F, P 100, RR 22, BP 120/70, Ht: 5'3", Wt: 260 lbs

General:	Responds only to deep pain
HEENT:	PERRLA, EOMI
	TMs clear
	Throat clear
Neck:	Supple
Heart:	RRR without murmurs, rubs, or gallops
Lungs:	CTA
Abdomen:	Bowel sounds present; no hepatosplenomegaly
Extremities:	No cyanosis, clubbing, or edema; **no** rash

Neuro: No focal neurologic signs

LABORATORY:

Lumbar puncture:
WBC: 110/mm^3; 50% neutrophils, 50% lymphocytes
RBC: 15 RBC
Protein: 80 mg/dL
Glucose: 67 mg/dL (plasma glucose 80 mg/dL)
Gram stain: Negative

CBC: Normal
Electrolytes: Normal
MRI of head: Focal lesion at the base of the left temporal lobe with mild edema
CXR: Normal

Which of the following is the most likely diagnosis?

A. Herpes simplex meningoencephalitis
B. Neurosyphilis
C. *Bartonella henselae* infection
D. Varicella meningoencephalitis
E. *Streptococcus pneumoniae* meningitis

576.

A mother brings her 3-year-old son to see you because he has been "falling down a lot." He's had no symptoms of illness. You start asking more questions, and you learn that he has been falling for the past few months and is getting progressively worse. He also has difficulty climbing stairs and gets up "funny" from sitting on the floor.

PAST MEDICAL HISTORY: He was born term without difficulty. He met all of his developmental milestones appropriately.

FAMILY HISTORY: Noncontributory

PHYSICAL EXAMINATION: Vital signs stable. He demonstrates hip girdle weakness and the Gower maneuver to rise from the floor to a standing position. Patellar reflexes are diminished.

LABORATORY: Creatine phosphokinase (CPK) is 20,000 IU/L (normal < 160 IU/L)
Muscle biopsy: Degeneration and variation in fiber size, deficiency of type IIB fibers and absent dystrophin.

Which of the following is the most likely diagnosis?

A. Becker muscular dystrophy
B. Spinal muscular atrophy
C. Duchenne muscular dystrophy
D. Myotonic dystrophy
E. Congenital muscular dystrophy

577.

Which of the following is the most common cause of chronic subdural hematomas in infants?

A. Scurvy
B. Child abuse
C. Biotin deficiency
D. Hemophilia
E. Congenital defects of the scalp

578.

You see a 1-year-old female whose problems began in infancy. Initially she began to develop hypotonia. Now she has progressed to the point where she has severe weakness. She has hyporeflexia on examination and muscle fasciculations are noted—particularly of her tongue. She has not had any seizures or fever.

Which of the following is the most likely diagnosis?

A. AIDS
B. Werdnig-Hoffman disease
C. Wilson disease
D. Medulloblastoma
E. Gaucher disease

579.

By what age should 90% of infants be able to <u>voluntarily</u> grasp a rattle?

A. 2 months
B. 4 months
C. 6 months
D. 8 months
E. 12 months

580.

On a neurologic developmental level, children are able to copy different shapes in a regular order.

Which of the following is the correct sequence in which children can copy these forms?

A. Square, cross, circle
B. Circle, cross, square
C. Square, circle, cross
D. Cross, square, circle
E. Circle, square, cross

581.

Which of the following is the average head circumference in the term newborn?

A. 30 cm
B. 25 cm
C. 35 cm
D. 40 cm
E. 45 cm

582.

A child can copy a circle and a cross for you but cannot copy a square.

Which of the following is her age likely to be?

A. 1 to 2 years of age
B. 5 to 6 years of age
C. 7 to 8 years of age
D. 2 to 3 years of age
E. 3 to 4 years of age

583.

At which age are 90% of infants likely to demonstrate a "social smile"?

A. Birth
B. 1 week
C. 2 weeks
D. 1 month
E. 2 months

584.

At which age are 90% of infants likely to demonstrate a "social laugh"?

A. 2 months
B. 3 months
C. 1 month
D. 6 weeks
E. 1 week

585.

At what age are 90% of children able to sit without support?

A. 10 months
B. 1 year
C. 5 months
D. 6 months
E. 7 months

586.

At what age can 90% of children walk unassisted?

A. 12 months
B. 7 months
C. 1 year
D. 14 months
E. 18 months

587.

At what age can the majority of children release an object into a hand?

A. 1 year
B. 8 months
C. 6 months
D. 4 months
E. 2 months

588.

At what age can most children walk up steps?

A. 2 years
B. 1 year
C. 14 months
D. 3 years
E. 16 months

589.

At what age can the majority of children "regard and reach for a raisin"?

A. 5 months
B. 8 months
C. 14 months
D. 2 months
E. 1 year

590.

Which of the following reflexes are normal in a newborn infant?

A. Moro reflex
B. Rooting reflex
C. Grasp reflex
D. Stepping reflex
E. All of the reflexes listed are "normal"

591.

All of the following are true about the "parachute" reflex except:

A. May persist for years.
B. A normal response is abduction and extension of the arms as if to break the fall.
C. It is normally symmetric.
D. Appears by 1 month of age.
E. An asymmetric response indicates hemiparesis or brain damage.

592.

Which of the following is true regarding the "Landau" reflex?

A. It occurs at the spinal cord level.
B. It is a spontaneous extension of the neck and spine with some stiffening of the lower extremities in response to being suspended prone by supporting the chest.
C. It appears at birth.
D. It persists till 10 years of age.
E. It would not be present in a normal 1-year-old.

593.

Which of the following is true with regard to the "crossed extension" reflex?

    A. It is a higher reflex.
    B. It is normally not present at birth.
    C. A positive response consists of flexion of the ipsilateral leg.
    D. It is a common finding in spastic cerebral palsy.
    E. It normally disappears by 2 weeks of age.

NEWBORN / PRENATAL CARE

594.

You are called to the newborn nursery to evaluate a male infant with yellow skin. The infant was born 20 hours ago to two Hispanic parents, following an apparently uncomplicated delivery. Mom's prenatal labs were unremarkable; she is blood type O positive. She was screened for group B strep and found to be negative. This male infant is the second child for her. She denies any problems with her firstborn, as well as any recent illness. The mother is breastfeeding and reports that she has not felt engorged. The nurses state the infant is sleeping normally and not particularly fussy. He feeds well if offered a bottle. The infant's vital signs are completely normal. Other than jaundice to the mid thorax, the infant's physical exam is completely normal.

Which of the following do you recommend?

A. Nothing because this infant has physiologic jaundice
B. Nothing because this infant has breast milk jaundice
C. A total bilirubin as well as CBC and blood cultures because this infant could be septic
D. A total bilirubin and CBC with smear and reticulocyte count to begin his workup for pathologic jaundice

595.

All of the following are true regarding phototherapy for neonatal jaundice <u>except</u>:

A. Blue-green wavelength light is most efficient in the conversion of bilirubin to lumirubin.
B. The greater the skin surface exposed, the more effective the phototherapy.
C. Intermittent phototherapy is more effective than that given continuously.
D. The closer the light source is to the infant, the more effective the phototherapy.

596.

You are called to the normal newborn nursery to evaluate a 4-hour-old infant with a bedside screening glucose of 23 mg/dL. This is the first child for this mother, who has poorly controlled gestational diabetes. Mom's medical history is otherwise unremarkable. Her prenatal labs were significant for a failed 3-hour GTT, but otherwise were appropriate. She has no family history of diabetes.

Upon exam, the infant's vital signs are normal, but the infant is quite jittery and weighs 4.5 kg. The nurses state that the infant refuses to feed. The rest of the physical exam shows marked adiposity but no other focal findings.

Which of the following is the most likely diagnosis?

A. Beckwith-Wiedemann syndrome
B. Transient neonatal hypoglycemia
C. Hypoglycemia in an infant of a diabetic mother
D. Neonatal diabetes mellitus

597.

You are called to the normal newborn nursery to evaluate a 4-hour-old infant with a bedside screening glucose of 23 mg/dL. This is the first child for this mother who has poorly controlled gestational diabetes. Mom's past medical history is otherwise unremarkable. Her prenatal labs were significant for a failed 3-hour GTT, but otherwise were appropriate. She has no family history of diabetes.

Upon exam, the infant's vital signs are normal, but the infant is quite jittery and weighs 4.5 kg. The nurses state that the infant refuses to feed. The rest of the physical exam shows marked adiposity but no other focal findings.

Which of the following is the best course of action?

    A. Repeat the glucose after a breast milk feed.
    B. Repeat the glucose after giving glucose water.
    C. Repeat the glucose 2 hours later.
    D. Send a confirmatory glucose to the lab and start an IV of dextrose in 10% water (D10W).

598.

You are called to the normal newborn nursery to evaluate a 4-hour-old infant with a bedside screening glucose of 23 mg/dL. This is the first child for this mother who has poorly controlled gestational diabetes. Mom's past medical history is otherwise unremarkable. Her prenatal labs were significant for a failed 3-hour GTT, but otherwise were appropriate. She has no family history of diabetes.

Upon exam, the infant's vital signs are normal, but the infant is quite jittery and weighs 4.5 kg. The nurses state that the infant refuses to feed. The rest of the physical exam shows marked adiposity but no other focal findings.

Within minutes, you recheck the glucose and begin IV D10W. The baby improves quickly after the IV begins.

Given this response, what does the future hold for this child?

    A. The infant is likely brain-damaged.
    B. The infant will likely develop juvenile diabetes.
    C. The infant is at increased risk for Type 2 diabetes.
    D. The infant will likely recover and do well.

599.

You are called at home about an infant that has just been delivered to a mom who is known to be a carrier of group B strep. She received a single dose of ampicillin approximately 1 hour prior to her delivery. Her OB felt that her precipitous delivery may have been caused by chorioamnionitis. The infant is ~ 20 minutes old, and the nurses tell you that his vital signs, including temperature, are normal.

Which of the following do you recommend?

    A. Observation in the nursery for the next 12 hours
    B. Full sepsis workup followed by close observation for the next 2 days
    C. Septic workup and IV antibiotics pending culture results
    D. Limited sepsis workup and rooming-in as the mother recovers

600.

You are called at home about an infant that has just been delivered to a mom who is known to be a carrier of group B strep. She received a single dose of ampicillin approximately 1 hour prior to her delivery. Her OB felt that her precipitous delivery may have been caused by chorioamnionitis. The infant is ~ 20 minutes old, and the nurses tell you that his vital signs, including temperature, are normal.

A septic workup is performed and IV antibiotics are begun pending cultures.

The blood cultures are sterile at 48 hours of age. The infant has fed well and has normal vital signs and a normal physical exam.

Which of the following would you do now?

    A. Continue antibiotics to complete a 7-day course.
    B. Discontinue antibiotics and discharge.
    C. Discontinue antibiotics and observe for another 24 hours.
    D. Continue PO antibiotics as an outpatient.

601.

You are called at home about an infant that has just been delivered to a mom who is known to be a carrier of group B strep. She received a single dose of ampicillin approximately 1 hour prior to her delivery. Her OB felt that her precipitous delivery may have been caused by chorioamnionitis. The infant is ~ 20 minutes old, and the nurses tell you that his vital signs, including temperature, are normal.

A septic workup is performed and IV antibiotics are begun pending cultures.

If the infant is found to have GBS septicemia, which of the following statements is true?

    A. He is likely to have GBS meningitis as well.
    B. He can be managed with oral antibiotics once sensitivities are known.
    C. He needs at least 7–10 days of parenteral antibiotics.
    D. Her future pregnancies are not at risk for GBS disease.

602.

Upon arrival in the neonatal intensive care unit, a term infant is noted to have a respiratory rate of 82 breaths/minute. His color is poor, capillary refill is delayed, and he is retracting and grunting with associated nasal flaring. He is noted to be tachycardic with a prominent apical pulse in the right lower sternal border. Bowel sounds are noted over the left chest, while breath sounds in the same area are markedly diminished.

Which of the following findings is most likely to be identified upon further evaluation of this patient?

    A. A scaphoid abdomen
    B. Hepatomegaly
    C. Low-set, small dysplastic ears
    D. Omphalocele
    E. Gastroschisis

603.

During initial evaluation of a 4-pound, 1-ounce female born at 36-weeks gestation, she is noted to have a head circumference of < 3rd percentile. Additional abnormalities include bilateral cataracts; multiple areas of scarring, some of which appear to follow along a dermatome; and a shortened hypoplastic left leg.

Which of the following is the most likely cause of the clinical findings in this patient?

    A. Cytomegalovirus
    B. Toxoplasmosis
    C. Varicella virus
    D. Herpes simplex virus
    E. An amniotic band

604.

A 22-year-old woman presents for her first prenatal appointment at 5-months gestation. She states she was unable to obtain earlier prenatal care due to "lack of insurance." She has a history of hypertension and has continued to take her antihypertensive medication along with an over-the-counter vitamin.

Which of the following medications is most likely to be associated with fetal abnormalities when taken during pregnancy?

    A. Methyldopa
    B. Labetalol
    C. Enalapril
    D. Nifedipine
    E. Hydrochlorothiazide

605.

A 7-pound, 1-ounce male infant is born at term to a woman with a history of severe postpartum depression following delivery of her first child. Throughout her most recent pregnancy, she took sertraline, 100 mg each day.

Which of the following symptoms during the newborn period is most likely related to antenatal exposure to a selective serotonin re-uptake inhibitor?

    A. Excessive lethargy
    B. Constipation
    C. Hyperglycemia
    D. Hyperthermia
    E. Tremors, jitteriness

606.

An 18-year-old female, who is at 24-weeks gestation, is found to have an elevated level of serum alpha-fetoprotein. An ultrasound reveals the presence of a meningomyelocele.

Which of the following medications, when taken during pregnancy, is most likely to be associated with these findings?

A. Valproic acid
B. Lithium
C. Sertraline
D. Levothyroxine
E. Montelukast sodium

607.

A 20-hour-old male infant is noted to have an increased respiratory rate associated with excessive secretions and drooling. During attempts at feeding, he frequently chokes and spits. Additional evaluation reveals that the infant has a tracheoesophageal fistula.

Which of the following anatomical configurations is most common?

A. Esophageal atresia with a distal tracheoesophageal fistula (Type C)
B. Isolated esophageal atresia (Type A)
C. Isolated tracheoesophageal (H-type) fistula (Type E)
D. Esophageal atresia with a proximal tracheoesophageal fistula (Type B)
E. Esophageal atresia with both a proximal and distal tracheoesophageal fistula (Type D)

608.

A male infant is born via emergency cesarean section, weighing 1.7 kg. His mother is a known prostitute and is HBsAg-positive.

Which of the following outlines the most appropriate immunization schedule for prevention of perinatal transmission of hepatitis B virus to this patient?

A. Administer hepatitis B vaccine (HBV) at birth, and at 1 and 6 months of age.
B. Administer HBV at birth, and at 1, 4, and 6 months of age.
C. Administer hepatitis B immune globulin (HBIG) at birth and HBV when the infant reaches 2 kg, followed by an additional dose of HBV at 1 and 6 months after the first dose.
D. Administer HBIG at birth and HBV at birth, and at 1, 2, and 6 months of age.
E. Administer HBIG and HBV at birth, and at 1 and 6 months of age.

609.

During an initial examination in the newborn nursery, a term female is noted to have a single umbilical artery. She has no dysmorphic features, her height, weight, and head circumference are all at or near the 45th percentile, and the remainder of her physical examination is unremarkable.

Which of the following should be included upon additional evaluation of this patient?

A. Cranial ultrasound
B. Renal ultrasound
C. Slit-lamp examination
D. AP and lateral radiographs of the chest
E. Direct laryngoscopy

610.

During examination of a 3-day-old infant just prior to discharge from the normal newborn nursery, a distinct and reproducible "jerking" sensation is noted during adduction of the left hip while posterior pressure is simultaneously applied.

Which of the following groups is at greatest risk of the disorder demonstrated by this clinical finding?

A. Boys with a breech presentation
B. Large for gestational age girls
C. Girls with a breech presentation
D. Large for gestational age boys
E. Girls with a positive family history of this disorder

611.

A 7-day-old female presents with a 2-day history of eye discharge. She was adopted at 2 days of age after her birth mother, who received no prenatal care, presented to the emergency room in labor. On physical exam, she has purulent discharge from both eyes. A direct fluorescent antibody (DFA) test on a conjunctival secretion specimen is positive for *Chlamydia*.

Which of the following potential complications is associated with the recommended treatment for this infection?

A. Generalized seizures
B. Pyloric stenosis
C. Hemolytic anemia
D. Hearing loss
E. Increased intraocular pressure

612.

Multiple cases of varicella are reported within an isolated rural community of families who shun routine immunizations for their children because of their religious heritage.

Assuming that permission is granted to proceed with treatment, which of the following individuals should receive passive immunoprophylaxis with varicella-zoster immune globulin following exposure to an index case?

A. A 10-day-old infant whose mother developed varicella one day earlier
B. An infant born at term whose mother developed varicella 3 days prior to delivery
C. A 5-day-old infant whose mother developed varicella one day earlier
D. An infant born at term whose mother developed varicella at 30-weeks gestation
E. An infant born at 33 weeks gestation whose mother developed varicella 2 weeks prior to delivery

613.

Twice within several hours, a 3-day-old female born at 33-weeks gestation is noted to have an intense period of reddening of a large portion of her skin, lasting for several minutes. During each episode, she was lying on her left side when she suddenly developed reddening on that side, which was clearly demarcated in a longitudinal fashion along her midline by a pale color covering the right side of her body. On each occasion, her color returned to normal after she was positioned on her back.

Which of the following is the most appropriate next step in the evaluation of this patient?

A. Abdominal ultrasound.
B. Evaluation of four extremity blood pressures.
C. Doppler ultrasonography of the renal veins and arteries.
D. Echocardiogram.
E. No further evaluation is indicated.

614.

A 39-year-old expectant mother has scheduled an appointment with you, because she has been advised by her obstetrician that her ultrasound shows she is pregnant with twins. She asks about care of twins and what special considerations she needs to keep in mind as she contemplates the delivery process. In particular, she seems concerned about breastfeeding and whether or not it is possible for her to do this.

What is your response to her regarding breastfeeding?

A. It is better to bottle feed to ensure that they receive adequate nutrition, due to concerns of low volume of breast milk initially.
B. Breastfeeding does not provide any benefit over bottle feeding.
C. One recommendation is to feed both infants at the same time, with one on each breast.
D. Most mothers of twins who choose to breastfeed realize it is too difficult.
E. If she supplements one of the babies with formula, it is a good idea to prop the bottle instead of holding it, so she can breastfeed the other child.

615.

The EDC (expected date of confinement) may be calculated by using various methods.

Which of the following statements is <u>not</u> true?

   A. In a woman with 28-day cycles, 280 days after the onset of the last menstrual period determines the EDC.
   B. That little wheel "thingee" can be used.
   C. Subtracting 3 months from the first day of the last menses and then adding 7 days determines the EDC.
   D. In women who use steroidal contraceptives immediately before pregnancy, the date of conception is easily calculated.
   E. In women with irregular menses, calculating the EDC is less precise.

616.

You are called to the delivery of a preterm infant whose mother has had no prenatal care. She presented to the hospital ready to deliver. By dates, the infant is 34-weeks gestational age. In the delivery room, the baby requires intubation and mechanical ventilation. After stabilizing the newborn, you complete your exam. You notice severe dilatation of the abdominal wall. Ultrasound demonstrates severe dilatation of the bladder resulting from urinary flow obstruction.

Which of the following is the most commonly associated anomaly found with this disorder?

   A. Unilateral cryptorchidism
   B. Low-set ears
   C. Bilateral cryptorchidism
   D. Microcephaly
   E. Micrognathia

617.

Which of the following is associated with gestational age less than 32 weeks?

   A. The ear has incurving of only the upper 2/3 pinnae.
   B. Lanugo is present only on the shoulders.
   C. Testes are in the upper scrotum.
   D. Labia majora is larger and nearly covers the clitoris.
   E. Smooth soles without creases.

618.

Which of the following is usually seen in a post-term infant and not a term infant?

   A. Hair is fine and woolly.
   B. Scrotum already has a few rugae.
   C. Dry, peeling skin and less than normal subcutaneous tissue.
   D. Abundant vernix.
   E. Lanugo only on the face.

619.

Which of the following is an abnormal finding on physical examination of a term newborn?

A. A spleen tip palpable at the left costal margin.
B. A liver tip palpable 2 cm below the right costal margin.
C. The labia majora meet at the midline and obscure the urethra and clitoris.
D. Penile length of 2 cm.
E. The lower portion of **each** kidney is palpable.

NUTRITION / TEETH

620.

You are seeing Amber Smith for her 12-month well-child checkup. Her mother reports that everything is going well except that Amber's appetite has drastically changed. For approximately the last month, she hasn't eaten nearly as much and some meals she won't eat at all. Amber's mother is offering a variety of nutritious foods for all 3 meals and 1 or 2 snacks per day. She has switched her to whole milk and is giving her the appropriate amount/day (12–16 oz/day).

PAST MEDICAL HISTORY: She was admitted for RSV at 6 months of age but otherwise has been very healthy. Immunizations are UTD. She is due for 12-month shots today.

On physical examination, her weight is at the 10th percentile (she was at the 25th percentile at 9 months). Length and head circumference are stable at the 50th percentile. Her physical examination is normal except she has a runny nose and congestion.

Which of the following would you tell her mother?

A. She should increase the number of snacks per day.
B. Since she's not eating, her mother should double the child's milk intake.
C. The child probably has food allergies and should see the allergist.
D. This is a normal phase, and she should continue offering a variety of foods without forcing the child to eat.
E. She should make Amber sit in her high chair until she eats everything on her plate.

621.

There are 9 essential amino acids that are not synthesized adequately and that humans require in their diets. However, 2 of these can be substituted with another amino acid.

Which of the following is a correct substitution pair?

A. Lysine by tyrosine
B. Histidine by tyrosine
C. Phenylalanine by tyrosine
D. Valine by tyrosine
E. Isoleucine by tyrosine

622.

We know that an individual's protein requirement varies with age.

Which of the following requires the highest protein requirement on a gram/kg/day basis?

A. The newborn infant
B. The adolescent having a growth spurt
C. A 6–12-month-old infant
D. A 4–6-year-old child
E. An adult

623.

Which of the following is the potential energy available from dietary fat?

A. 3 kcal/g
B. 9 kcal/g
C. 5 kcal/g
D. 4 kcal/g
E. 2 kcal/g

624.

Which of the following is true about cholesterol?

A. Cholesterol is the principal dietary sterol.
B. Cholesterol is available from exogenous dietary sources.
C. Cholesterol is available from endogenous sources.
D. Dietary changes in cholesterol intake will result in only minor changes in total plasma cholesterol.
E. All of the choices are true.

625.

Which of the following is not observed with essential fatty acid deficiency?

A. High levels of linoleic acid
B. Reduced growth velocity
C. Scaly dermatitis
D. Increased susceptibility to infection
E. Decrease in arachidonic acid levels

626.

There are marked changes in total body water (TBW), intracellular water (ICW), and extracellular water (ECW) concentrations in children as they age from birth to adulthood.

Which of the following is true regarding body distribution of water in a 10-year-old compared to an infant at birth?

A. TBW decreases, ICW decreases, and ECW decreases.
B. TBW increases, ICW increases, and ECW increases.
C. TBW decreases, ICW increases, and ECW decreases.
D. TBW increases, ICW increases, and ECW decreases.
E. TBW decreases, ICW decreases, and ECW increases.

627.

Carol Berk is a 3-month-old, 5-kg infant who has been having severe diarrhea for 3 days. She has the following physical findings: tenting of the skin, depression of the anterior fontanelle, tachycardia, and oliguria. She has normal blood pressure and capillary refill is < 3 seconds. You estimate her fluid deficit at 10%.

Which of the following is the correct amount of fluid resuscitation that she will require?

A. 1,500 mL of 5% dextrose IV, to which 40 mEq of potassium chloride and 57 mEq of sodium is added
B. 500 mL of 5% dextrose IV, to which 40 mEq of potassium chloride and 57 mEq of sodium is added
C. 1,200 mL of 5% dextrose IV, to which 40 mEq of potassium chloride and 57 mEq of sodium is added
D. 2,000 mL of 5% dextrose IV, to which 40 mEq of potassium chloride and 57 mEq of sodium is added
E. 1,000 mL of 5% dextrose IV, to which 40 mEq of potassium chloride and 57 mEq of sodium is added

628.

James Brown is an 8-year-old child who normally weighs 25 kg. He has been having diarrhea and vomiting for several days. You estimate that he has a 5% fluid deficit.

How much fluid resuscitation over 24 hours would be needed to return him to baseline?

A. 1,700 mL
B. 2,850 mL
C. 1,250 mL
D. 1,600 mL
E. 2,250 mL

629.

A 2-month-old infant weighs 5 kg and has 5% dehydration. Her serum sodium returns at 120 mEq/L. You calculate that she needs 750 mL of water over the next 24 hours.

Based on her sodium deficit, how much sodium should be added to this 750 mL of fluid?

A. 45 mEq
B. 60 mEq
C. 100 mEq
D. 81 mEq
E. 86 mEq

630.

A 2-month-old infant weighs 5 kg. She has developed severe dehydration. She comes in with a serum sodium of 168 mEq/L. Based on this you know she has a hypertonic dehydration.

What is her total 24 hour requirement of fluid, and what amount of this is required to be given as "free water"?

A. 1,000 mL total, 175 mL "free" water
B. 1,500 mL total, 175 mL "free" water
C. 1,000 mL total, 100 mL "free" water
D. 1,000 mL total, 300 mL "free" water
E. 1,200 mL total, 300 mL "free" water

631.

Which of the following is recommended for exclusively breastfed infants?

A. No supplementation is necessary regardless of the water source.
B. If the mother lives in a community with fluoridated water, no supplementation is necessary.
C. Folate supplementation.
D. Fluoride supplementation.
E. Vitamin E if the child lives in high sunlight exposure areas of the United States.

632.

Infants fed human milk or infant formula not fortified with iron should start to receive a dietary source of iron by what age?

A. From birth
B. 2 months of age
C. 6 months of age
D. 1 year of age
E. Not necessary until 2 years of age

633.

What is the primary role of 1,25 (OH)$_2$D?

A. Stimulate absorption of calcium and phosphorus from the stomach.
B. Stimulate absorption of calcium and phosphorus from the small intestine and reabsorption of calcium from the kidney.
C. Stimulate absorption of calcium and phosphorus from the large intestine and reabsorption of the calcium from the kidney.
D. It has no function except to be a prohormone for vitamin D.
E. It stimulates excretion of parathyroid hormone.

634.

Which of the following is a contraindication to enteral tube feeding?

A. Coma
B. Severe cardiac abnormalities
C. Incompetent lower esophageal sphincter
D. Pancreatitis
E. Necrotizing enterocolitis

635.

Natal teeth usually erupt in which position in the mouth?

A. Lower molar position
B. Upper incisor position
C. Lower incisor position
D. Upper molar position
E. Lower canine position

636.

Which of the following is the proper sequence for the eruption of teeth?

A. Maxillary central incisors, mandibular central incisors, second molars
B. Mandibular central incisors, maxillary central incisors, second molars
C. Mandibular central incisors, second molars, maxillary central incisors
D. Maxillary central incisors, second molars, mandibular central incisors
E. Second molars, maxillary central incisors, mandibular central incisors

637.

By 1 year of age, most children have how many deciduous teeth?

    A. 1 to 2
    B. 2 to 4
    C. 6 to 8
    D. 12 to 14
    E. 6 to 8 plus 2 permanent teeth

638.

A 7-year-old comes in with an autosomal dominant disorder (her father has this same condition). The crowns of her teeth have normal form and size but are translucent blue to dark gray, with an opalescent sheen. A biopsy is done and shows that the dentin is dysplastic with dentinal tubules that are irregularly arranged and sometimes absent. The roots from one extracted tooth are extremely short. She has no enamel left on any of the older teeth, although a tooth that is now erupting still has enamel on it. Her father's teeth are worn down to the gingival margins.

Which of the following is the most likely diagnosis?

    A. Hurler's syndrome
    B. Ellis-van Creveld syndrome
    C. Cherubism
    D. Hallermann-Streiff syndrome
    E. Dentinogenesis imperfecta (hereditary opalescent dentin)

639.

The first permanent teeth to erupt are usually which of the following?

    A. Central incisors
    B. Lateral incisors
    C. First molars
    D. Second molars
    E. Premolars

RESPIRATORY

640.

A 10-year-old African-American male presents to your office for further evaluation of his persistent wheezing. He was referred from the emergency room where he has been seen twice this year. He required a 5-day course of oral steroids with each visit. His only medications are albuterol in both MDI and nebulized forms. He relates that he has cough and/or wheeze approximately 2–3 times a week, usually associated with moderately vigorous exercise. He also awakens from sleep due to his asthma once a week and requires his inhaler. Physical exam in the office is normal. Office spirometry shows a FEV_1/FVC of 76%.

Based on the NHLBI Expert Panel Report 3 (EPR3) asthma guidelines, which of the following best classifies this patient?

A. Mild intermittent
B. Mild persistent
C. Moderate persistent
D. Severe persistent

641.

Based on the NHLBI EPR 3 asthma guidelines, the most preferred first step in therapy for moderate persistent asthma would be which of the following?

A. Short-acting beta agonists
B. Low-dose inhaled corticosteroids
C. Low-dose inhaled corticosteroids and long-acting bronchodilator
D. High-dose inhaled corticosteroids and long-acting bronchodilator

642.

A 2-week-old female presents to your office for a checkup. Results from newborn screening revealed elevated immunoreactive trypsinogen (IRT) and two copies of the delta F508 mutation.

As you begin to discuss the diagnosis of cystic fibrosis with this family, what can you tell them based on the mutational analysis?

A. This child will most likely have severe lung disease.
B. This child will most likely have pancreatic insufficiency requiring oral enzyme supplementation.
C. This child will most likely be infertile.
D. This child will most likely have learning disabilities.
E. Nothing, because this child does not have cystic fibrosis.

643.

A Caucasian male weighing 3.1 kg and estimated to be 38-week gestation developed respiratory distress requiring intubation and mechanical ventilation shortly after birth. He had no other congenital anomalies. Pregnancy and delivery were uncomplicated, and the mother received appropriate prenatal care. Attempts to wean the infant off the ventilator are now unsuccessful after 4 weeks. ECHO is normal. The infant has no signs of infection. CXR shows a diffuse interstitial pattern.

Which of the following would be the next best step in the evaluation?

    A. Sweat test
    B. Evaluation for immune deficiency
    C. Referral for lung transplant
    D. Lab test for surfactant deficiency

644.

Which of the following children should receive treatment for tuberculosis?

    A. A 6-year-old with cough, negative CXR, PPD 3 mm, and who has a cousin that was recently diagnosed with TB.
    B. An asymptomatic 10-month-old, mother recently diagnosed with TB (now on therapy), negative PPD, and CXR showing right lower lobe peripheral infiltrate.
    C. A 3-year-old with negative CXR, negative PPD, and classmate's mother recently diagnosed with TB.
    D. All should be treated.
    E. None should be treated.

645.

A 3-year-old female presents for evaluation of chronic cough. The cough has been present for the past 6 months. It is worse when she first awakens and anytime she is lying down. The parents have noted significant halitosis upon awakening. They deny that she has had any fever or headaches. She has had no wheezing. The cough usually sounds productive but they have seen no sputum. They deny rhinorrhea but have noted nasal congestion intermittently. On exam, the child has normal lung auscultation.

Which of the following would be the most appropriate therapy?

    A. Initiation of inhaled corticosteroids
    B. Trial of proton pump inhibitor
    C. Antitussive therapy
    D. Initiation of antibiotic therapy for 3–4 weeks

646.

A 6-month-old female presents to the emergency room for respiratory distress. The mother relates she had recent upper respiratory symptoms and now has rattling in the chest. On auscultation, the child has expiratory stridor. Past medical history is unremarkable. No history of choking or aspiration. No chronic cough. She has shown good weight gain. CXR and CT chest are below:

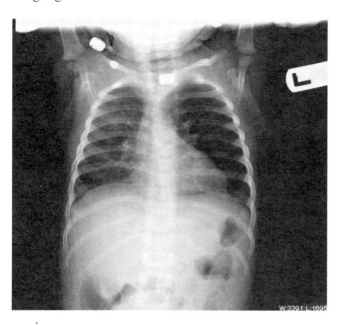

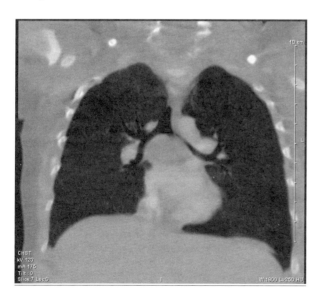

Based on these findings, which of the following is the best next step?

A. Observation
B. Open lung biopsy
C. Removal of lesion surgically
D. Fungal serologies

647.

A 10-year-old female with HIV presents to clinic and is noted to have tachypnea, mild retractions, and crackles on auscultation. The mother states the child has been eating poorly and is less active than normal. No fever or upper respiratory symptoms are noted. CT chest shown below reveals diffuse interstitial process.

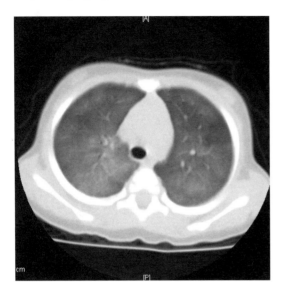

Which of the following is the most likely etiology?

    A. Bronchiolitis obliterans
    B. Lymphoid interstitial pneumonitis
    C. Usual interstitial pneumonitis
    D. Desquamative interstitial pneumonitis

648.

Which of the following proposed mechanisms of action best describes the potential benefit of racemic epinephrine in bronchiolitis?

    A. Racemic epinephrine reduces microvascular leak and airway edema.
    B. Racemic epinephrine decreases viscosity of airway mucous.
    C. Racemic epinephrine stimulates receptor in airway muscle to increase contractility.
    D. All of the answers are correct.

649.

Which of the following is (are) seen in patients with sickle cell having acute chest syndrome?

    A. Bradycardia
    B. Pleural effusions
    C. Hemoptysis
    D. Pulmonary infiltrates

650.

Which of the following is the most common reason for the development of obstructive sleep apnea in preschool age children?

A. Obesity
B. Congenital airway anomalies
C. Tonsillar and adenoid hypertrophy
D. Decreased central respiratory drive

651.

In a patient with scoliosis, cardiopulmonary compromise occurs in which of the following cases?

A. There is no compromise regardless of degree of curvature.
B. If there is a greater than 45 degree curve.
C. There is compromise at any degree of curvature.
D. If there is a greater than 90 degree curve.

652.

Which of the following factors is associated with a poor prognosis in a drowning event?

A. Age less than 2 years.
B. Water temperature is less than 10° C.
C. It takes more than 30 minutes before life support is begun at the scene.
D. Resuscitation takes longer than 25 minutes.

653.

A 12-year-old female with a history of moderate persistent asthma presents for routine follow-up. At the time of her initial visit, you prescribed low-dose inhaled steroids and a leukotriene modifier. She reports that since her initial visit, she has had minimal daytime symptoms. She has required her rescue inhaler only 2–3 times a week and awakens from sleep only about 3–4 times a month. She reports that, overall, she feels the medications are working great. She denies significant exercise limitation. She has had no exacerbations requiring oral steroids or acute intervention by another physician (such as an emergency room, acute care, etc.).

Based on the history provided by the patient, you would classify her control as which of the following?

A. Well controlled
B. Not well controlled
C. Very poorly controlled
D. Unable to assess based on this information

654.

A 37-week-gestational male is born and immediately begins to experience respiratory distress. Physical exam reveals a scaphoid abdomen and decreased breath sounds in the left chest.

Which of the following statements is true about this diagnosis?

    A. The herniated intestine is more likely to occur on the right.
    B. Mortality is related to the size of the diaphragmatic defect.
    C. The most common site of herniation is a posterolateral defect.
    D. The infant will develop pulmonary hyperplasia on the same side as the defect.

655.

A 5-year-old female is referred to you. She was recently tested for alpha-1-antitrypsin (α1-AT) deficiency because of family history. She was found to have a PI_{ZZ} phenotype with an α1-AT level of 20.

Which of the following is the most likely clinical manifestation that would be seen at this age?

    A. Hepatic manifestations
    B. Recurrent pneumonia
    C. Emphysema
    D. Diarrhea

656.

Which of the following statements is correct regarding cystic fibrosis (CF)?

    A. All patients are pancreatic insufficient.
    B. A positive newborn screen is diagnostic for CF.
    C. All patients are infertile.
    D. Nutritional status is strongly correlated to pulmonary status.

657.

In the workup of recurrent pneumonia, the single most valuable piece of information is which of the following?

    A. Prior growth chart
    B. CBC obtained at the time of most recent pneumonia
    C. Prior chest radiographs
    D. Results of sputum culture

658.

A 15-year-old female with a negative past medical history presents for evaluation of recurrent chest pain. She describes this pain as sharp, localized (midsternal), and not associated with nausea or diaphoresis. She states that when the pain occurs, it is worse with inspiration but relieved within a few minutes of onset. There have been no identified triggers, and pain can occur with exertion or at rest. On auscultation, the lung fields are clear and no murmur is appreciated. Pulmonary function tests are also normal.

Which of the following is the test that will most likely result in a diagnosis?

A. Obtaining a 12-lead ECG
B. Obtaining a chest radiograph
C. Palpation of the costochondral junctions
D. Measurement of oxygen saturation pre- and post-exercise

659.

Which of the following is the most common complication of acute upper respiratory infection in children?

A. Otitis media
B. Sinusitis
C. Asthma exacerbation
D. Pneumonia

660.

A 14-year-old male living in the Chicago area presents with fever, chills, productive cough, and pleuritic chest pain. In review of his recent history, he reported that he had gone with his family on a camping trip to the Chain O'Lakes State Park three weeks prior to presentation. Sputum culture was obtained and showed the following:

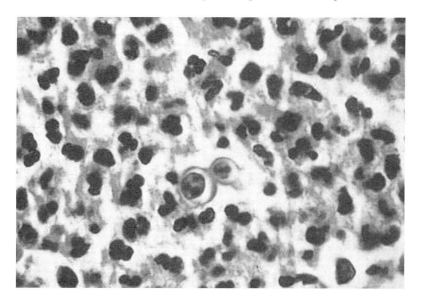

Which of the following is the most likely diagnosis?

    A. Histoplasmosis
    B. Nocardiosis
    C. Blastomycosis
    D. Coccidiomycosis

661.

A 9-month-old boy presents with a 3-week history of cough associated with posttussive vomiting. A polymerase chain reaction (PCR) assay from a nasopharyngeal specimen is positive for *Bordetella pertussis*.

Which of the following outlines a recommended treatment for household or other close contacts of this patient?

    A. A 9-month-old who has received 3 DTaP vaccines who attends the same day care center in the same room as the index patient should receive a 4th DTaP.
    B. Only those day care attendees who are not up to date with DTaP immunizations should receive chemoprophylaxis.
    C. All daycare attendees should receive chemoprophylaxis regardless of immunization status.
    D. All household contacts under the age of 7 years should receive a DTaP immunization if their last DTaP vaccine was a year or more earlier.
    E. Chemoprophylaxis is only indicated when < 10 days have elapsed since the onset of cough in the index patient.

662.

A 3-month-old boy presents to the emergency room because his parents noted that he "was coughing so hard he turned blue and vomited." He has a 2-week history of cough and congestion. The cough has continued to worsen and is now so frequent that he is having difficulty breastfeeding. He coughs frequently during examination and on one occasion, coughs continually for a period of 15–20 seconds and is noted to become cyanotic.

Which of the following findings is most likely to be identified upon further evaluation of this patient?

    A. An elevated WBC count with a predominance of lymphocytes
    B. A prominent consolidation on chest x-ray in the right middle and right lower lobes
    C. Elevated liver function tests
    D. Evidence of widespread retinal hemorrhages on examination of the fundi
    E. A vesicular rash most prominent on the anterior and posterior trunk

---

663.

An 11-year-old malnourished boy presents with a history of frequently falling when running or climbing stairs. He was recently placed into a foster home after being removed from his biological parents due to medical neglect. Both parents were subsequently incarcerated for substance abuse and trafficking drugs. The patient's only complaint is that his feet "always feel like they are asleep and burning." His foster parents state that they were informed by a social worker that the patient was to continue to take isoniazid, which he began several months earlier, because "he had been around people with tuberculosis and had a positive skin test."

Which of the following is the most likely cause of this patient's symptoms?

A. Pyridoxine (vitamin B_6) deficiency
B. HIV/AIDS
C. Drug-induced hepatotoxicity
D. Thiamine (vitamin B_1) deficiency
E. Cobalamin (vitamin B_{12}) deficiency

664.

A 26-month-old girl presents to the emergency room with a 2-day history of "cough and wheezing." Her parents also report that she appears to become "short of breath" with only minimal activity. Her past medical history is positive only for recurrent episodes of wheezing that usually were associated with an upper respiratory infection. Her parents also report progressive hoarseness. On physical examination, she is afebrile. Her respiratory rate is 38. Her breathing is labored and she has biphasic stridor. She has a clear nasal discharge, is not drooling, and appears well hydrated. A radiograph of the neck shows a soft tissue irregularity at the vocal cord level.

Which of the following is the most likely cause of this patient's findings?

A. *Haemophilus influenzae type b*
B. Parainfluenza Type 2 virus
C. Human papillomavirus subtype 6
D. *Staphylococcus aureus*
E. *Streptococcus pyogenes*

665.

A 3-month-old boy is hospitalized because of continued worsening of upper respiratory symptoms, including a prominent cough associated with posttussive vomiting. During evaluation, a polymerase chain reaction (PCR) assay for *Bordetella pertussis* is positive.

Which of the following additional laboratory findings is most likely to be identified in this patient?

A. An elevated WBC count associated with an increased percentage of segmented neutrophils
B. An elevated WBC count associated with an increased percentage of eosinophils
C. A depressed WBC count associated with an increased percentage of segmented neutrophils
D. An elevated WBC count associated with an increased percentage of lymphocytes
E. A depressed WBC count associated with an increased percentage of lymphocytes

666.

The parents of a 2-year-old girl present to the emergency room with concerns that their daughter "is having difficulty breathing." She is able to sit calmly with her mother. Her temperature is 101.2° F and her respiratory rate is 28. Her voice is hoarse, and she is noted to have inspiratory stridor when crying. There is no evidence of associated cyanosis. Capillary refill is < 3 seconds. Examination of her lungs reveals numerous transmitted upper airway sounds.

Which of the following is most likely to be identified during radiographic evaluation of this patient?

   A. Consolidation of both upper lobes on chest x-ray
   B. Increased soft tissue width in the retropharyngeal space on lateral roentgenogram of the neck
   C. Swollen epiglottis on lateral roentgenogram of the neck
   D. Pseudomembrane detachment in the trachea on lateral roentgenogram of the neck
   E. Subglottic narrowing on chest x-ray

667.

A 3-week-old infant presents with a history of worsening cough. Her mother reports difficulty with feeding and episodes of posttussive vomiting. Paroxysms of cough are observed during physical examination, and the patient is admitted for additional evaluation. The patient is subsequently diagnosed with pertussis.

Which of the following represents a potential complication of treatment in this patient?

   A. Infantile hypertrophic pyloric stenosis (IHPS)
   B. Toxic megacolon
   C. Intussusception
   D. Volvulus
   E. Achalasia

668.

A mother brings her 18-month-old daughter to see you for a cough that started approximately 3 hours earlier. It's a hard, dry cough, and she can't seem to stop. She's had no fever or cold symptoms. She has been healthy except for 1 episode of RSV at 8 months of age, which did not require hospitalization.

On physical examination, the patient is coughing off and on. Ears, nose, and throat are clear. Lungs have diffuse wheezes on the right with decreased air movement. Clear on the left with good air movement. RR 40. No stridor.

You obtain a CXR that shows hyperinflation on the right side. No other abnormalities noted.

Your treatment plan includes which of the following?

   A. Referral for rigid bronchoscopy
   B. Albuterol and inhaled steroids
   C. Decadron
   D. Racemic epinephrine
   E. Albuterol plus oral steroids

669.

All of the following are true regarding the mechanisms of action of inhaled glucocorticoid therapy <u>except</u>:

A. Inhibition of cytokine production
B. Inhibition of inflammatory cell recruitment
C. Inhibition of mediator release
D. Decreases microvascular leak therefore decreases edema formation
E. Down-regulation of beta-adrenergic receptors

670.

Which of the following is a normal respiratory rate for a 1-year-old child?

A. Over 55 breaths/minute
B. Between 20 and 30 breaths/minute
C. Between 10 and 20 breaths/minute
D. Between 30 and 40 breaths/minute
E. Between 10 and 12 breaths/minute

671.

A 13-year-old girl had influenza A diagnosed last week. She comes in today with much worsening of her cough and return of her fever. She was feeling better near the end of the week but now, in the last 24 hours, has become acutely ill again. She says that she has pain in her left lower chest when she takes a deep breath. Before this influenza diagnosis, she has been healthy.

PAST MEDICAL HISTORY: Negative
                                      Took amantadine for 5 days; finished 3 days ago

SOCIAL HISTORY: Doesn't smoke but exposed to 2nd hand at home—her mom smokes

FAMILY HISTORY: Non-contributory

REVIEW OF SYSTEMS:
    Fevers to 103° F
    Chills
    Sore throat now resolved
    Body achiness is severe again

PHYSICAL EXAMINATION:
BP 110/70, P 80, RR 24, Temp 102° F
Ill-appearing girl in moderate distress

    HEENT: PERRLA, EOMI;
                    TMs clear
                    Throat slightly hyperemic
    Neck: Supple, no masses
    Heart: RRR without murmurs, rubs, or gallops

Lungs:	Diffuse crackles fairly localized to the left base
Abdomen:	Bowel sounds present; no hepatosplenomegaly
Extremities:	No cyanosis, clubbing, or edema

Laboratory: is pending

Besides *Streptococcus pneumoniae*, which other organism should you consider in this patient?

A. *Staphylococcus aureus*
B. *Haemophilus influenzae*
C. *Streptococcus pyogenes*
D. *Staphylococcus epidermidis*
E. *Mycoplasma pneumoniae*

672.

A 6-year-old child has been on mechanical ventilation for one week due to ARDS, which was contracted from a pneumococcal pneumonia. She is slowly being weaned. Clinically, she is doing well and you are pleased with her progress.

MEDICATIONS: Day 8 of Ceftriaxone

Objective data from today:

HEENT:	Pupils responsive and equal
	Mild thrush of her oral mucosa
Neck:	Supple, no masses
Heart:	RRR without murmurs, rubs, or gallops
Lungs:	Still with basilar crackles right greater than left
Abdomen:	Positive bowel sounds, tolerating tube feeds well; no masses
Extremities:	No cyanosis, clubbing, or edema

LABORATORY:

CBC shows a mild increase in WBC to 11,000 from 9,500 yesterday with 80% lymphs
Sputum culture from 2 days ago returns today and shows *Pseudomonas aeruginosa* sensitive only to amikacin, piperacillin/tazobactam, and ceftazidime

AST: 25
ALT: 26
Bilirubin: 0.2 mg/dL
Creatinine: 0.5 mg/dL
BUN: 10 mg/dL

CXR: Mild improvement from admission; no new infiltrates

Based on your information from today, what would you do at this point?

A. Switch antibiotic coverage to piperacillin/tazobactam alone.
B. Add amikacin to ceftriaxone.
C. Switch antibiotics to piperacillin/tazobactam + amikacin.
D. Continue current therapy.
E. Perform bronchoscopy and then start piperacillin/tazobactam + amikacin.

673.

Which of the following is <u>not</u> considered an indication to place a patient on treatment for latent tuberculosis infection (assume all CXRs are normal)?

    A. PPD reading at 72 hours of 7 mm of a patient on 5 mg/day of prednisone
    B. PPD reading at 72 hours of 11 mm in a prisoner
    C. PPD reading at 48 hours of 6 mm in a patient who lives with a person who has active tuberculosis
    D. PPD reading at 48 hours of 16 mm in a healthy 13-year-old
    E. PPD reading at 72 hours of 11 mm in a diabetic

674.

You are seeing a 17-year-old boy who lives on a farm and has a herd of cattle. About 3 weeks ago, he was helping a cow deliver and had to assist the cow by manually removing the calf and the placenta. The cow was well before the delivery. Your patient became ill about 2 days ago with a high fever, night sweats, and cough. He has noted that he also has left upper quadrant tenderness in his belly.

PAST MEDICAL HISTORY: Negative, healthy farm boy

SOCIAL HISTORY:
                 Lives with his mother, a widow woman
                 Has 3 cats, 2 dogs, and a pet iguana
                 Chews tobacco
                 Doesn't drink alcohol

FAMILY HISTORY:
                 Dad died at the age of 35 in a bull riding accident
                 Mother healthy, 40-years-old
                 Has 2 younger sisters

REVIEW OF SYSTEMS:
        Complains of joint aches and pains with the fever
        Headache
        Weakness

PHYSICAL EXAMINATION:
BP 110/80, P 110, RR 20, Temp 103° F, Ht 6'1", Wt 210 lbs
Well-developed, very muscular boy in some distress

      HEENT: PERRLA, EOMI
                   TMs Clear
                   Throat: mild erythema
      Neck: Supple, no meningismus
      Heart: RRR without murmurs, rubs, or gallops
      Lungs: Coarse breath sounds with defined crackles at the right base
      Abdomen: Bowel sounds present; liver down 5 cm below right costal margin; spleen tip
                   down 4 cm below left costal margin
      Extremities: No cyanosis, clubbing, or edema
      Skin: No rashes

LABORATORY:

WBC: 18,000/mm^3; 75% polys, 20% bands

Hgb: 16.0 mg/dL

Platelets: 150,000

Electrolytes are normal

AST: 100

ALT: 120

CXR: Right lower lobe pneumonia

Which of the following is the likely etiology of his pneumonia?

A. *Francisella tularensis*
B. *Streptococcus pneumoniae*
C. *Staphylococcus aureus*
D. *Coxiella burnetii*
E. *Yersinia pestis*

Question 125:

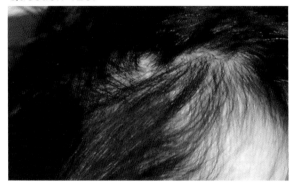

Question 128:

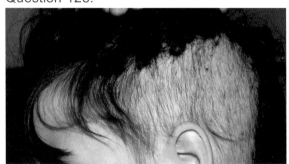

Question 130:

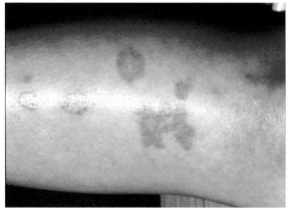

Question 131:

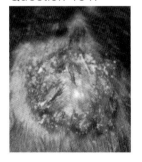

Question 133:

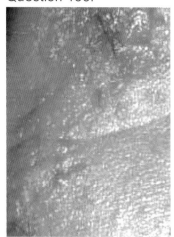

Question 135:

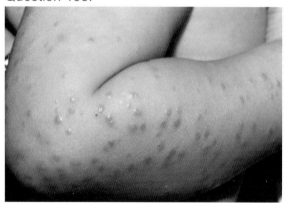

Question 137:

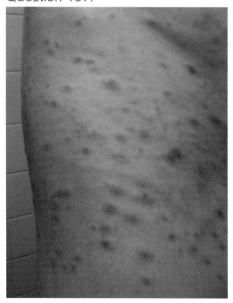

Question 141:

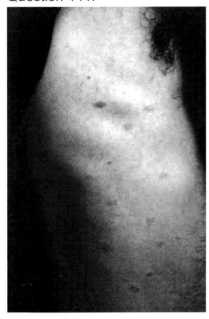

Question 145:

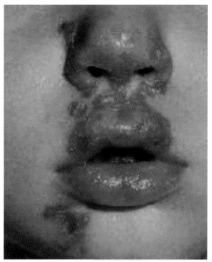

Question 142:

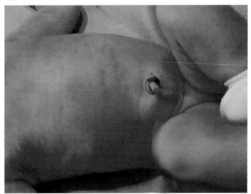

Question 149:

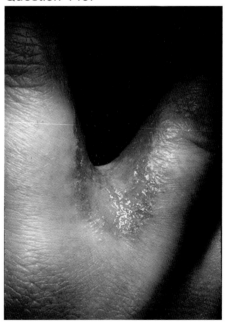

Question 144:

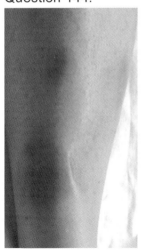

Question 150:

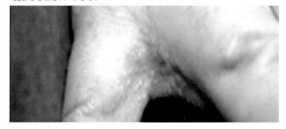

Question 151:

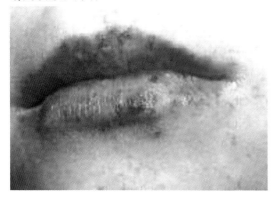

Question 153:

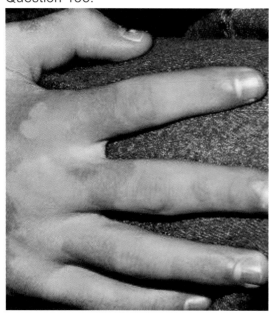

Question 456:

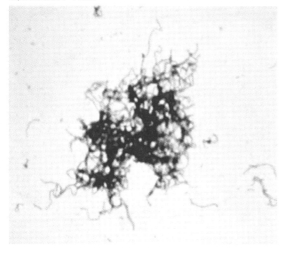

Question 489:

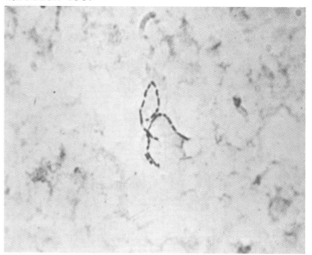

Question 493:

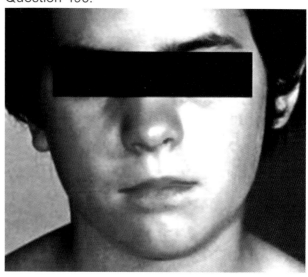

Question 501:

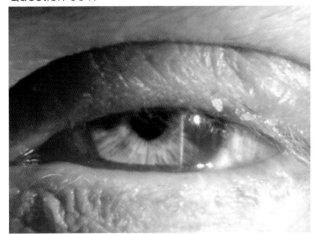

Question 557:

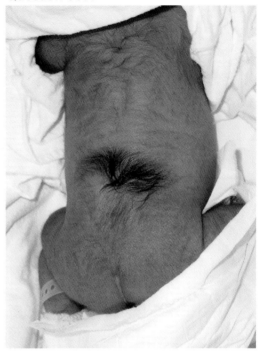

Question 551:

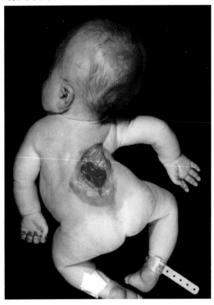

Question 660:

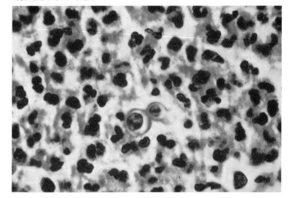